# Therapeutic Nursing and the Hospitalised Elderly

## Alison L. Kitson

DPhil, BSc (Hons)(NUU), RGN

Dissertation submitted for the degree
of Doctor of Philosophy from the
School of Social Sciences of the University of Ulster

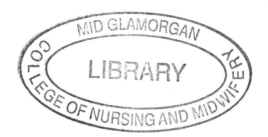

ROYAL COLLEGE OF NURSING
RESEARCH SERIES

Scutari Press

**Aims of the Series**
To encourage the appreciation and dissemination of nursing research by making relevant studies of high quality available to the profession at reasonable cost.

The RCN is happy to publish this series of research reports. The projects were chosen by the individual research worker and the findings are those of the researcher and relate to the particular subject in the situation in which it was studied. The RCN in accordance with its policy of promoting research awareness among members of the profession commends this series for study but views expressed do not necessarily reflect RCN policy.

# Scutari Press
Viking House, 17–19 Peterborough Road,
Harrow, Middlesex HA1 2AX, England

A subsidiary of Scutari Projects, the publishing company of the Royal College of Nursing

First published 1991

**British Library Cataloguing in Publication Data:**
Kitson, Alison L.
  Therapeutic nursing and the hospitalised elderly.
  1. Old persons. Nursing
  I. Title  II. Series
  610.7365

  ISBN 1-871364-27-2

Typeset by Action Typesetting Ltd., Gloucester
Printed and bound in Great Britain by
Billing & Sons Ltd, Worcester

# Contents

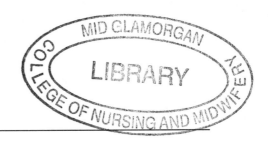

'For us who nurse, our nursing is a thing which, unless in it we are making progress every year, every month, every week, take my word for it, we are going back.'

*Florence Nightingale (1914)*

# Acknowledgements

I should like to thank the Department of Health and Social Services of Northern Ireland for funding the first two years of this research project through a nursing research studentship, and also Age Concern for sponsoring the final two years of study. Help from all grades of nursing stafff throughout the Province must also be acknowledged, not only for their co-operation and assistance in providing information and filling in rather formidable questionnaires, but also for allowing me the privilege of spending time with them and learning from them. Sincere thanks must also be extended to colleagues in the Nursing Studies Department, and members of other departments in the University of Ulster, whose experience, knowledge, wisdom and advice were greatly appreciated. Finally, I would like to thank my family and friends, who tolerated months of relative neglect from a daughter, wife and friend.
Thank you.

Alison L. Kitson

# Summary

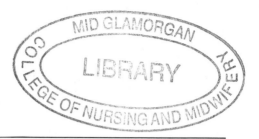

The study of geriatric nursing sought to explain why a minority of nurses gave patient-centred care while the majority were content to provide care that was routine-oriented and depersonalised. The influence of the medical model was not considered to be solely responsible for the nursing profession's apparent inability to ensure a better quality of care. Rather, the proposition was that the nursing profession had not clarified its position in relation to the care of the elderly and, in consequence, could offer little guidance and direction to those who worked in geriatric wards. This was the result of nursing's failure to accept care as its central function, to identify the main components of caring for the hospitalised elderly and to develop a geriatric nursing model to organise, control and direct nursing practice.

The explanation of why some nurses gave personalised care whereas the majority gave poor care was felt to rest with the nurse's understanding of her primary function. The components of care were identified by constructing a theoretical model based on Norton et al's (1962) innovative work and supplemented by Orem's (1980) concepts of self-care. This model became the means by which good nursing care could be recognised from poor nursing care. The instruments that were constructed to achieve this included the TNF Indicator and the TNF Matrix. The TNF Indicator sought to distinguish those ward sisters who were aware of their therapeutic nursing function from those who were not. A social survey approach was used to test the indicator on a randomly selected group of ward sisters across Northern Ireland. Two groups emerged: one with a positive approach to the care of the elderly, the other manifesting a more routine approach. These findings were validated by a detailed study of the quality of nursing care in three wards. The therapeutic content of patients' self-care activities, which was measured by the TNF Matrix, was found to be better in wards whose sister had a high TNF score than in wards where the ward sister had a low TNF score. Neither improved environmental facilities nor increased medical and paramedical involvement affected the therapeutic content of patients' self-care activities.

Thus, ward sisters who were aware of their therapeutic function were found to organise their work and approach patient care in a manner similar to that of the activities outlined in the theoretical framework. The TNF Indicator identified aspects of organisational ability, knowledge and attitudes towards care, whereas the TNF Matrix acted as a quality of care indicator. Through the theoretical framework and the instruments that were developed, a more precise model of geriatric care could be constructed that would ensure that the qualities of a few staff are transmitted to the majority, in order to improve the standard of care for the hospitalised elderly.

# 1 | Concepts of geriatric care

In tracing the development of geriatric nursing care from its roots in Poor Law institutions to its present day structure, it is necessary to consider two concepts that have influenced nursing action. These are, first, the extent to which nursing has identified its central caring function in society and, second, a consideration of the philosophy of geriatric care.

## PARAMETERS OF THE CARING FUNCTION

### Personal and moral characteristics

The concept of care is fundamental not only to the nursing profession but also to the whole system of interdependent relationships that characterise the mutual support and aid given within a family or within a community setting. Griffin (1983) has described caring as a fundamental concept, both in the philosophy of human nature and in that of personal relationships. Caring denotes a primary mode of being that fashions and directs human relationships; it requires a personal commitment or measure of involvement characterised by prolonged and reliable attention. Caring also requires a moral obligation from the carer to provide a service that is acceptable to the recipient of that care.

Both the personal and moral characteristics of the caring function can be transposed onto a wider social setting. A caring society – or a caring community – is one in which the needs of individuals are served by others' concern and protection of them (Tinker, 1981). The so-called 'caring professions' should, therefore, comprise those groups whose direct responsibility would be to construct a system to ensure such services.

1

In general terms, the concept of care can be described as involving both the servicing of individual needs and concern for and protection of others. Griffin (1983) has further identified two distinct areas: first, the moral responsibility to care, which comprises such activities as 'interest', 'attention', 'consideration', 'guidance' and 'service' and, second, the personal inclination to care. Incorporated in the latter are the more emotive considerations such as liking someone, being attached to someone and wanting to be near someone.

A further cluster of meanings relates to attitudinal aspects of the individual faced with some form of reciprocal caring relationship. In such a situation, cognitive, moral and emotional factors come together to play a significant part in the form that the caring activity takes. In terms of nursing, the outworking of such an activity is seen in what happens between the nurse and the patient, in the activities that are performed and in the attitudes and feeling underlying them. The notion of a caring relationship also has temporal and spatial aspects (Bergman, 1983), which demand from the care-giver a more or less long-term disposition to act and feel in certain acceptable ways.

Thus, while performing a basic nursing function in providing an element of care for another individual, the nurse undertakes both moral and personal duties. She may perform her task competently and with skill but without personal involvement.

## Emotional aspects

It is Griffin's (1983, p.291) belief that when the nurse performs activities without expressing particular emotions or displaying more personal attributes of the caring function, it cannot be called caring. She further states that the recipient of care has a right to demand emotional care because, as a human being, respect and dignity of person are deserved.

Griffin continues:

> 'The patient's predicament (being ill) illuminates that essential humanity under threat and is thus a profound call for the attention of the giver of care: a protector of humanity. The attempt to understand another person then centrally requires that we understand that person's emotional life; his wants, desires and priorities.'

Griffin identifies some qualities of the carer as they are perceived in nurse–patient relationships, in which the carer not only provides competent physical care but also is aware of the patient's emotional needs. These qualities include the ability of the nurse to reflect upon the patient's particular situation and to be mature enough to become aware of the other person's needs. It is in the nurse's ability to perceive and judge each particular situation that the wide array of helping activities that constitutes caring is seen as being grounded. Furthermore, in being able to give her attention afresh to each situation, the nurse displays the ability to attune herself to the commonplace. Once identified, the patient's need is met by nursing action that may encompass several strata: the clinical assessment, cognitive and moral recognition of the patient as a person and, finally, the emotional element of the act.

The significance of the emotional aspects of caring has also been described by Hirschfeld (1983) and Bergman (1983). In a study that explored the factors influencing the care-giver (in this case a family) to continue living with and caring for an old person with irreversible senile brain disease, Hirschfeld (1983) found that it was in those situations in which a mutually reinforcing relationship existed between the dependant and the carer that the patient was cared for and coped with at home. More significantly, in situations where low mutuality or no mutuality existed between carers and dependants, Hirschfeld reported that the relationship was in jeopardy of disintegrating under the strain. It would seem, therefore, that the emotional aspects of caring provide not only greater incentive and meaning for the carers but also the means for coping with more difficult situations.

Bergman (1983) illustrates this when she describes a situation where an elderly lady suffering from senile dementia was pacified by the actions of a nurse who perceived the patient's emotional needs and reacted in such a way as to pacify her. The nurse's action comprised sitting on the patient's lap, putting her arms round her and hugging and kissing her. The reaction of the patient, Bergman reports, was that she relaxed and became calm, having found a haven of familiar security.

Such a concept of care, however, may involve potential dangers for the nurse by becoming over-involved with the patient's situation, thus making herself more vulnerable. This could be countered by providing the correct supportive framework within which the nurse–patient relationship can develop. Bergman (1983) sees professional autonomy and responsibility for the nurse as integral components of this framework, which, by providing the necessary guidance and support, would be responsive to the physical and emotional stress inherent in the nurse's caring function. Yet within this system, the patient would still occupy the central position.

**Caring as a shared role**

Besides the emotional aspect of the nurse's caring function, there is a further important characteristic of the concept of care that has a significant impact on the nature of nursing. McFarlane (1976) referred to this when she stated that although the caring role is central to nursing, it is nonetheless shared with patients themselves, their relatives and other health professionals. From a nursing point of view, care is both a central and a shared role, and the nurse, therefore, must be aware of her interchangeable role in caring for her patients. The nature of the nurse's actions will be determined not only by the particular needs of the patient, but also by the ability and availability of other professional and lay carers.

McFarlane does not see the interchangeability of the professional and non-professional roles as a threat to the nurse's unique function, which is embodied in the provision of activities of daily living to individuals who are unable to provide such care for themselves. A more difficult situation is one in which nursing itself devalues those activities that have come to be known as basic nursing care. Both McFarlane (1976) and Henderson (1980) have commented on the grave conceptual and practical problems resulting from this devaluation of the nurse's caring function. In an article that examines the essence of nursing, Henderson (1980, p.246) points out that although there is an overlapping of nursing with many other health-care fields, nurses do have a unique function, namely to help persons, sick or well, from birth to death, to carry out those activities of daily living that they would perform unaided if they had the strength, the will and the knowledge. Throughout this relationship, nurses help people to live independently and, when independence is impossible, to cope with disability and, finally, to die with dignity. Henderson concludes by saying that the essence of nursing – basic nursing care – is essential to human welfare.

McFarlane (1976) refers to Henderson's (1966) concept of nursing as well as Orem's (1971) definition, in which nursing is identified as an act of assisting or helping someone who is unable to help himself in activities related to self-care. This type of care, which she terms primary nursing, is seen as involving the nurse in professional action and independent function. McFarlane uses five general methods of giving help or assistance identified by Orem (1971). Such helping methods range from providing total help by acting and doing for another, through guiding, supporting and providing a therapeutic environment, to teaching another. McFarlane feels that nursing practice has concentrated on the first method of helping, at the expense of the development of the other aspects of the nurse's skill repertoire.

Linked with the nurse's failure to define her primary caring role with clarity, and to develop it, is the tendency of society at large to confer greater value upon the 'curing function' than that of 'caring'. Indeed, it may be that the public's stereotyped image of the nursing function is linked more to the nurse's ancillary curing role. The potential danger of this misrepresentation has been identified by McFarlane (1976), who feels that the nurse's talent for caring, helping and assisting may be overlooked by the nursing profession and, as a result, given over to unskilled workers, while nurses concentrate on becoming 'technicians'.

Ironically, it would seem that the most basic element of human existence, i.e. one's need of care, has been undervalued as an activity by the nursing profession. Rather than concentrate on the challenge of providing care to those who are dependent on help to perform basic activities of daily living, nurse training and skills have focused on the medical model. Nursing's lack of understanding of its caring function is perhaps best demonstrated in the contradictions it faces in those areas in which cure is an impossible goal and care is the central focus, e.g. the long-term care of elderly infirm.

## Totality of care

So far, the discussion has considered the main elements of the concept of care as it relates to nursing. These have included suggestions that caring is a universal task that is provided personally, by professionals, or by a community. Caring activities also embrace moral and personal elements, which manifest themselves in the form of helping actions and attitudes towards the emotional needs of the person requiring care. Nursing is seen as synonymous with caring (Henderson, 1966, 1980; Griffin, 1980;

Bergman, 1983), and yet, regrettably, confusion seems to exist in the mind of the profession and of society as to the real nature of nursing. Often, it is the medically oriented model of nursing care that captures the public's imagination, to the demise of the nurse's caring function.

Perhaps it was in defiance of this stereotype that Norton (1965, p.51) claimed it was geriatric nursing that was 'the sensitive index by which to measure nursing's standards of care since it is nursing, undiluted and unadorned'. If geriatric nursing is to be the measure by which the profession gauges its success, nursing's standards of care still leave much to be desired. Recent studies of nursing care of the hospitalised elderly (Baker, 1978; Miller, 1978; Wells, 1980; Evers, 1981a) demonstrate how nursing has yet to take seriously its responsibility of being the major caring profession. Some might argue that nursing's failure to define clearly its caring role is related to the presence of a burgeoning and oppressive medical model, which has stressed active care and recovery (Evers, 1981b). Others (Towell, 1975; Baker, 1978) blame both the profession and the social system that disadvantages the elderly, further devaluing them when they are faced with the double indignity of being old and disabled.

It is the argument of this thesis, however, that the major responsibility for the poor state of geriatric nursing care lies with the nursing profession. Despite early attempts at identifying and developing a framework for geriatric nursing care (Norton et al, 1962; Norton, 1965), very little progress has been made towards understanding and expanding the nurse's unique contribution in the care of the elderly. While medical and social care of the elderly were developing theoretical frameworks that delineated and defined each practitioner's sphere of professional responsibility (Brocklehurst, 1978; Jeffreys, 1978), nursing seemed content to replace the rigid ward routines of bedside nursing care with equally rigid routines of chairside care of the elderly infirm (Norton, 1977). Given the scope and challenge of providing care to elderly persons, one must ask why this was allowed to happen.

## CONCEPTS OF GERIATRIC CARE

Although the term geriatrics, from a combination of the Greek words 'geron' (old man) and 'iatreia' (treatment), was first used by Nascher in 1909 to describe the care of illness in old age, it was not until the late 1940s that the term was used to describe the care of the elderly infirm within the British health-care system. The term was seen to represent a change in the attitudes surrounding the treatment and care of the elderly, from a system based in the repressive and custodial attitudes of the Poor Law to one of a positive approach to the treatment and care of the elderly infirm (Norton, 1977).

This change came about as the result of the rising proportion of old people in the population and the increasing demands they made on the social and health-care services (Adams and Cheeseman, 1951). Between 1907 and 1945 the elderly population of Great Britain more than doubled, from around 2.5 million to nearly 7 million (Tinker, 1981). This rise produced not only a volume increase in the demand for services but also a growing awareness of the need to provide services tailored to the particular needs of the elderly.

MacIntyre (1977) has argued that the ideological change from a custodial model of care to a more humanitarian model, as exemplified in the philosophy of geriatric care, had more to do with pragmatism than altruism. The institutional model of care was incapable of coping with the growing numbers of elderly infirm, thus necessitating an alternative approach to the problem.

In addition, the advent of the National Health Service brought to the proper notice of the hospital authorities the inequalities that had been tolerated within the two hospital systems – the acute and chronic sick sectors. The advances that had been realised in the acute hospital sector served only as all too obvious reminders of the social and medical neglect of the need of the chronic sick and elderly.

Thus, linked with the geriatric care philosophy that old people deserve and require a better service than that which they are offered by the old dual hospital system was the commitment to provide better facilities that would link the general and chronic sick wards (Adams, 1960). The geriatric unit was the embodiment of this idea – a unit which, according to Adams (1960, p.815):

'sought to eliminate physical disability or reduce it as much as possible, and to retrain the patient to live and to work within the limits of his disability but to the hilt of his capabilities.'

Another feature of geriatric care, acknowledged at this time, was the close link between social and health-care provision. Studies by the Rowntree Committee on the problems of ageing and the care of old people in the 1940s, together with health-care studies of the elderly in the community (Sheldon, 1948), served to underline the need for a co-ordinated approach to providing an adequate service. Recognition of this feature is seen in the structure of the geriatric care team, which comprises a range of community and hospital health and social service workers.

Nursing care provision was also altered by the new concept of geriatric care. Norton (1977, p.1622) had emphatically stated that the nursing of old people is not geriatric nursing unless it contains the practice of the positive approach to the health and welfare problems of old people. Theoretically, this philosophy has been translated into nursing action by replacing routinised bedside care with more individualised care, in which the nurse's actions are determined by her assessment of the elderly person's need for assistance rather than by the ward routine.

The design of ward facilities and the provision of suitable equipment have also been identified as essential ingredients in the provision of geriatric nursing care (Adams, 1960; Norton et al, 1962; Norton, 1967, 1970). Adams states:

> 'We believe the success or failure of the work of a geriatric unit depends so much on the nurses that they should have the best possible facilities for their work.' (p.815)

Thus, the essence of geriatric nursing care is linked with a positive attitude to the care of the elderly, the reorganisation of routines of care and the restructuring of the ward environment. The aim of this is to enable elderly people to 'maintain or regain the maximum enjoyment compatible with their acquired pathology for the remainder of their lives' (British Geriatric Society, 1976). This aim comes close to the definitions given of the nurse's caring role in which her duty is to provide assistance with those activities of daily life that the individual is incapable of performing for himself.

In order to look more closely at how the major health-care professionals accepted and internalised the concepts of geriatric care, the main characteristics of geriatric medical care and geriatric nursing will be considered.

## Geriatric medical care

Social and medical commentators are agreed that the origin of health care for the elderly was based on the social organisation of care for those in the community who were unable to care for themselves – the poor, the sick, the elderly, the unemployed. Brocklehurst (1978) has described the history of care for the elderly as emerging from the Poor Relief Act of 1601, by which the community was charged with responsibility to care for its dependants. In the nineteenth century, society's responsibility for the elderly infirm was discharged in the principles and philosophy of the Poor Law Amendment Act of 1834, by which the health-care needs of such individuals were often subsumed under a heavier yoke of social deprivation due to the status of the inmates of the Poor Houses.

Elsewhere, Brocklehurst (1975) describes the effect of the development of the dual hospital system on the care of the elderly, stating that it was not until the state took responsibility for the large numbers of chronic sick beds in the public hospital system that the real needs of the elderly were recognised. Examples of the types of patient who were to be found in the old chronic sick wards were described by Adams and McIlwraith (1963). They identified four distinct groups: the first group, 'the recovered', consisted of a few active people, recovered from illness, who were social misfits retained to help in the short-staffed wards; the second group comprised homeless people, disabled to some extent but capable of self-care; the third and largest group was the long-stay invalids; whereas the final group was made up of a small number of patients who seemed capable of response to further treatment.

Accurate classification and diagnosis of patients' medical conditions and recovery potential were the foundation stones of the new approach to geriatric medical care. A further guiding principle of the service was that it based its approach on the acute medical model of care, namely the problem-solving approach to illness, characterised by diagnosis and treatment, with the goal being cure and discharge of the patient (Hodkinson, 1981; Coakley, 1982; Horrocks, 1983). The distinctive features of such an approach, which has been widely advocated and described by geriatric medical specialists (Adams, 1960, 1964; Exton-Smith, 1962; Brocklehurst, 1978, 1975), have all been developments of the basic medical model. Figure 1 illustrates how the main medical

| Traditional medical model | Geriatric medical model |
|---|---|
| Diagnosis | • Pre-admission assessment (recognition of social factors in treatment and care of elderly)<br>• Altered reactions of illness in old age<br>• Treatment of acute or chronic conditions |
| | *The assessment/acute ward* |
| Treatment | • 'Traditional' treatment – therapeutics/surgery<br>• *Rehabilitation* of patients – medical personnel aided by team of paramedical workers<br>• *Treatment at day hospital* – elderly patients are allowed more time to regain their strength/optimal functional capacity |
| | *The rehabilitation ward* |
| Cure | • Goal of cure accomplished in patients who are discharged at a level of independence similar to that which they enjoyed prior to their illness<br>• Successful cure/recovery in elderly also depends on community support and family involvement |
| *Discharge/supervision – alternative arrangements for those who do **not** respond – long-term care* | |

Figure 1 The geriatric medical model

features of the present geriatric service have developed from the medical model of care.

Features of the geriatric medical model that make it operational include:

• the concept of progressive patient care;
• the concept of team work;
• the concept of geriatric medicine as a medical specialty.

*Progressive patient care*
The concept of progressive patient care was established early on in the evolution of the geriatric medical model approach to the needs

of the hospitalised elderly. Its development was in response to the distinctive needs of three main groups of patients, namely assessment, rehabilitation and long-stay patients. Assessment patients comprise those elderly infirm who require thorough medical examination and access to acute diagnostic facilities. Patients normally stay in such wards for 2 to 3 weeks, being discharged if fully recovered or being transferred to rehabilitative care.

Rehabilitation wards, which normally service one third of all patients admitted to acute wards, are responsible for the provision of paramedical and nursing facilities (Brocklehurst, 1975). The objective is to provide support and to help the patient to regain control of his disabled limbs and bodily functions. The average length of stay on rehabilitation wards is approximately 3 months, in which time over half those patients being treated are discharged, whereas approximately one quarter find themselves in the third stage of progressive patient care – long-term care.

The average length of stay in long-term care facilities is approximately 3 years (Hodkinson and Hodkinson, 1981). Patients are those who:

'despite the fullest application of medical treatment and attempts at rehabilitation fail to make a sufficient improvement to allow their return to the community and need care in hospital for the rest of their life.' (Hodkinson 1981, p.46)

Long-stay wards are usually situated in small, local hospitals rather than in the main district general hospital, the implication being that such patients are beyond medical reclaim. This geographical isolation has certain benefits but also potential dangers. The benefits of providing separate ward facilities for long-stay patients have been strongly advocated by Brocklehurst (1978), whereas Hodkinson (1981) is more cautious about the potential harmful effects of geographical separation in relation to standards and staff morale.

The physical separation of the geriatric medical function into assessment, rehabilitation and long-stay care wards reflects quite distinctive operational goals and models of care. Both the acute and rehabilitation wards may be seen to follow the orientations and goals of the traditional medical model – the achievement of high patient turnover, treatment and cure of patients. The final stage of the progressive patient care model, however, tends to be more problematic in accommodating itself to the acute care goals.

An alternative interpretation of the progressive patient care concept is the division of one ward into acute, rehabilitation and continuing care sections. This approach was advocated by Adams (1964), who feared that if those patients in the largest and most vulnerable section of geriatric medicine – the long-stay patients – were separated from the geriatric unit, it could herald the development of a second-class system of geriatric care. Thus, by making each ward responsible for at least 40% long-stay patients, Adams believed that standards of care would adhere to the philosophy of providing a positive approach to care of the elderly. Brocklehurst (1978) and Hodkinson (1981), however, have argued that this approach may be more for the convenience and morale of nursing staff than in the interest of the patients.

Regardless of whether progressive patient care is practised over several facilities or within one ward, it can be said that the principles involved reflect the acute medical model approach – making full use of diagnostic services and treatment facilities and having as one's goal successful recovery and discharge until proven otherwise. These themes are found not only in the medical texts describing the organisation and philosophy of geriatric care but also in current government documents on health care of the elderly, e.g. *The Way Forward* (Department of Health and Social Security, 1977) and *A Happier Old Age* (Department of Health and Social Security, 1978).

## Teamwork

In his introductory text on geriatrics, Hodkinson (1975, p.2) says, 'Geriatrics is clearly concerned with the whole patient'. He describes geriatric medicine as being responsible both for the general medical care of the elderly and for rehabilitative, psychiatric and gerontological aspects of their care.

In a similar vein the British Geriatric Society and the Royal College of Nursing document (1975, p.31) states:

> 'Old people may suffer from a variety of illnesses, physical, psychological and social, at one and the same time, therefore professional staff with different knowledge and skills can be involved in diagnosis, treatment and care.'

The document goes on to outline the need for close communications and co-operation, the sharing of information and expertise and the election of a strong and appropriate team leader, if teamwork is to be successful. A recent study (Evers, 1981b) on the effectiveness of teamwork questions, however, the whole premise on which the notion of teamwork and interprofessional co-operation is based. Evers contends not only that teamwork in geriatric care is often a myth but also that it may have particularly undesirable consequences for long-stay patients and nursing staff.

Evers argues that the goals enshrined in the concept of teamwork are linked with the overall goals of the geriatric medical model of care, which focus primarily on diagnosis and treatment of assessment and rehabilitation patients. Other workers are co-opted to help in the process, particularly in the rehabilitation stage when recovery is prolonged. The notion of teamwork is accepted in situations where the diagnosis and treatment follow predictable medical model patterns, but, says Evers, when there is a more difficult case, a non-conformer to the treatment model, the inadequacies of the team concept are highlighted.

Evers exemplifies this by describing the experience of two elderly patients who were 'non-conformers'. Both patients' care required more than a straight medical solution, but the appropriate 'specialists' in the team were not encouraged by the medical staff to initiate any more radical solutions. This is perhaps one of the most pertinent dangers of linking the teamwork concept too closely with the geriatric medical model, in that it is unable to meet the complex needs of the irremediable or long-stay patients.

## A medical specialty

Strengthened by the demographic changes that will place even more importance on the medical care of the elderly, the profession must consider how geriatric medicine will develop in the future. These developments will also indicate the priorities and objectives of such a service.

Pathy (1982) has identified three broad operational concepts that would affect the future shape and orientation of geriatric medical care. These are the practice of geriatric medicine without acute or assessment patients, the treatment of a clearly defined range of acute conditions that fall within prescribed limits, and the provision of a broad service to meet the needs of all those people over 75 years of age, whether suffering from acute or chronic conditions.

From a professional medical point of view, the first two options would seem to be least attractive, in that the prized goals of the acute medical model – treatment and cure – would be difficult to obtain. Adoption of a geriatric service concentrating on long-term care would require reorientation of the aims and goals of the geriatric medical model. Fears of the return to a custodial care approach have been voiced by the medical profession when either of these options has been mentioned (Evans et al, 1971; Hodkinson and Jeffreys, 1972).

The model of choice for the future development of the speciality of geriatric medicine appears to be the age-related option. Not only would the goal of treatment and cure be realised more often in this model but also the continuity of treatment and cure would be more adequately assured. According to Horrocks (1979, p.263):

> 'A commitment to an age group is much more acceptable in terms of status to many hospital staff than is a commitment to a disease process or to a severe degree of disability. The attractiveness of geriatric medicine is inevitably reduced if the geriatric department is seen by those not working exclusively with the elderly as a repository only for patients deemed too distasteful, too disabled or too difficult for their own wards.'

Government and policy documents similarly emphasise the importance of acute and rehabilitative care for the hospitalised elderly. The government document, *A Happier Old Age* (Department of Health and Social Security, 1978, para 7.4) states that an active approach to treatment of the elderly 'can only be satisfactorily achieved in a general hospital, where the full range of diagnostic and therapeutic facilities are available and where there is adequate and suitable rehabilitation provision to assist recovery'.

*The Way Forward* (Department of Health and Social Security, 1977) recommends greater use of hospital beds, in terms of increased throughput. Both the profession's view, as reflected in documents such as the British Medical Association report *Care of the Elderly* (1976) and the Royal College of Physicians report (1977), and the Government's attitude would be sympathetic to the view that geriatric medicine is best implemented through a modified acute medical model whose goal is accepted, either implicitly or explicity, as cure. Problematic to this approach is the position of the long-term care patient whose goal is not cure but a prolonged need for care. It is to the development in this aspect of geriatric care, as it relates to the nurse's function, that attention will now be focused.

### Geriatric nursing care

The main objective of this section is to consider how the concept of geriatric nursing care has been interpreted by the nursing profession. The previous sections have described how the acute medical model was redefined to provide a more positive method of medical treatment and care for the hospitalised elderly. In the same manner, attempts will be made to identify an equivalent nursing care model on which the principles of geriatric nursing care rest.

While it has been argued that many of the improvements in the care of patients within the Poor Law institutions and workhouses of the nineteenth century were attributable to the development of nursing as a profession (Abel-Smith, 1960; White, 1978; Baly, 1980), nurses cannot claim to be the pioneers of the concept of enlightened care of the chronic sick and elderly infirm. Rosemary White (1978) states that the Poor Law nurses became the first geriatric nurses. This view can only be accepted if they were seen to adopt and adhere to the new positive approach to geriatric care. Geriatric care was attempting to replace a policy of custodial care, in which patients who had not conformed to medical expectations of recovery and discharge were accommodated in an environment governed by routines and regulations and in which the nurse's duty was to provide 24-hour bedside care (Norton, 1977).

The lack of importance attached to the chronic sick by the medical profession was also reflected in the attitudes of the nursing profession. Writing in 1954, Norton described how, in order to change the approach to nursing the elderly sick, two things were essential:

> 'first to re-educate those with old and established ideas that all the patient needs is toilet attention and feeding, and secondly, to educate the rising generation of nurses to the scope and interests of the work.' (p.1253)

Nursing care of the elderly, however, was not part of the student nurse syllabus, and this was the case until 1973 (Reid, 1981). This omission has helped to reinforce the false dichotomy between basic nursing and technical nursing (McFarlane, 1976), the former being associated with unskilled, basic nursing care and the latter embodying the well-accepted stereotype of the general nurse, skilled in the management and care of the acutely ill.

The development of the assistant nurse grade in the early 1940s (Abel-Smith, 1960; Baly, 1980), as a supplement to the decreasing numbers of state registered nurses willing to work in the chronic sick wards, also reinforced the division in the mind of the profession between the skilled and unskilled, the acute and chronic areas. The resultant image of the nurse working in a geriatric ward was of someone with no nursing qualifications who may have been sent to the ward as punishment for having committed some misdemeanour, or someone who was seen as unfit for a proper nursing post in the more acute wards (Rands, 1972; Norton, 1977).

It was into such an arena that the philosophy of geriatric care was placed, spearheaded by a more radical medical approach to diagnosis, treatment and care of the chronic sick. One of the first effects on nursing care was the shift in emphasis from bedside to chairside nursing care. Norton (1977, p.1623) described the impact of such a management shift without adequate explanation of the accompanying philosophy or objectives as both tragic and traumatic: tragic in the sense that nurses changed one routine for another without due reflection, and traumatic in that 'the whole foundation of nursing practice was shattered, all techniques, procedures and routines having been evolved from care of the patient in bed'.

*The impact of the medical model*
With the introduction of progressive patient care, nurses working in the new geriatric wards were being required not only to care for acutely ill patients but also to distinguish between methods of helping rehabilitation patients and to provide continuous, supportive care for long-stay patients. The ward environment had also changed; diagnostic and screening facilities, along with adequate rehabilitation facilities, met the medical needs of elderly patients, while more profound changes had to be made to the ward environment in order to meet the nursing care goals of providing an environment that would stimulate and encourage independence – the provision of adequate 'living space' for patients and suitable toilet, bathroom, dining-room and day-room facilities.

Thus, the nursing profession was having to cope with several major changes in the treatment and care of elderly patients imposed on it by the medical profession while it continued to find meaning for its own actions from the deeply ingrained, custodial care attitudes that had directed and given meaning to the care of the elderly infirm. The dilemma facing nursing was how to provide a meaningful framework of geriatric nursing care to replace the custodial model, that had dictated and given meaning to nursing action. Having identified a suitable geriatric nursing care framework, the new philosophy would provide practice guidelines for nurses working in the new geriatric wards. The challenge to nursing was to establish the position of the nursing care of the elderly as a legitimate and worthy task in no way secondary to acute nursing care and, at the same time, to identify the specific characteristics of geriatric nursing care.

## A geriatric nursing care model
As in the claims of McFarlane (1976) and Henderson (1980) that nursing's primary function is to care for and meet the basic self-care needs of individuals, Norton (1965) argues that it is in meeting the basic self-care needs of the elderly sick that the essence of nursing is experienced. Indeed, she claims that it is the nursing care of irremediable patients that is true nursing, 'where people of medical science hold but a watching brief while nursing really comes into its own' (Norton, 1965, p.58).

Norton's declaration of the central importance of meeting the basic self-care needs of the elderly in the development of her concept of geriatric nursing care is an important feature. The commonly accepted model of nursing care, fashioned for the care of acutely ill patients, is based on concepts such as the execution of medical directions and meeting the dependency needs of patients nursed in bed. In chronic sick wards, where the medical input is minimal, the traditional role of the nurse has been to meet the total dependency needs of the patient. Nursing goals were achieved when patients were 'clean, comfortable and contented' and had 'pressure areas intact' (Norton, 1981).

In order to safeguard against such attitudes, the first principle of the geriatric nursing care model accepts the central importance of care as nursing's primary function (Norton, 1965). The second important principle, outlined by Norton and later stated by the British Geriatric Society Memorandum (1976), is that geriatric nursing care is to adopt a 'positive approach to the health and welfare problems of old people'. The nurse's contribution to providing positive care is envisaged as distinct from, but complementary to, the geriatric medical function. Thus, the geriatric nursing care model would have elements in it reflecting the impact of the geriatric medical model, but yet would be distinctive in its own right.

## Basic elements of the geriatric nursing care model

One of the first geriatric nursing texts to appear, written by Rudd (1954), was called *The Nursing of the Elderly Sick*. This book stands out as an important landmark in the development of geriatric nursing as a speciality, and provides a succinct description of the aims and objectives of geriatric nursing care.

Early on, Rudd outlines the aims of nursing care of the elderly as including the maintenance of physical, mental and social independence, the prevention of chronic ill health and the maintenance of the individual in the community rather than in an institution.

He goes on to say that the provision of a purely custodial approach to long-term illness has been replaced by investigation, medical treatment and mobilisation. The results of this are greater teamwork, better prognosis and more effective treatment of such common symptoms as confusion and incontinence. Rudd adds:

> 'These fundamental changes in attitude are leading to a re-defining of the role of the nurse who is now being clearly seen as being concerned with the *total needs of the individual and the restoration of function rather than merely his temporary nursing requirements.*' (p.26, emphasis added)

Norton et al (1962) further identified important aspects of the nurse's function in the care of the elderly sick. Among other things, their study dealt with the organisation of nursing on geriatric wards, where they identified the need to provide a nursing care system that meets the individual needs of the elderly patient *within* the geriatric medical perspective of progressive patient care. Norton et al identified three major nursing care problems that were inhibiting a more positive approach to geriatric nursing care. These were the lack of accurate records of the nursing needs of the patient, no accurate nursing assessment of patients' capabilities and, finally, a routine approach to patient care, which was determined by the time of day and the geographical layout of the ward.

In order to overcome these nursing care problems, Norton et al suggested the assessment and subsequent grouping of patients in the ward according to *nursing requirements*. The need for individual nursing records for each patient was also emphasised, being seen as an essential step towards identifying and thus attempting to solve specific nursing problems. These records would also improve communication between carers, ensuring continuity of treatment regimens.

The main features of a geriatric nursing care model identified by Norton et al include: the need for individualised patient care, based on an accurate assessment of each patient's abilities followed by the identification of the patient's nursing needs; the need for systematic study of basic nursing care activities, e.g. the provision of nourishment, daily hygiene, meeting patients' elimination needs, etc.; the recognition of the importance of the environment as a potential nursing tool in terms of the ward design, furniture and equipment; and, finally, the need to consider the *total needs* of individual patients and to set *realistic goals* for each patient.

The relationship between the geriatric medical and nursing models is also considered by Norton (1965), who describes geriatric nursing as being made up of two distinct groups. She identifies the first group as assessment and rehabilitation patients or, in nursing terms, 'those patients who have a potential to regain the ability of basic self-care' (Norton, 1965, p.60). The second group of patients are those who have gone beyond medical reclaim and need some degree of nursing care for the remainder of their lives – the long-stay category.

The nurse's function for the first group of patients is in the 'reablement of the basic elements of self-care' – helping the elderly person to feed, wash, dress and get to and from the lavatory unaided. Norton (1965) identifies the range of nursing skills as including the ability to withdraw nursing care in such a way that the nurse, instead of 'acting and doing for the patient', learns how to support, encourage, supervise and teach the patient. The nurse also has to learn how to work in a team whose goal is the rehabilitation or reablement of the patient.

In the care of irremediable patients, the nurse's primary function is to 'maintain the delicate balance between giving of tender loving care and the maintenance of the last vestiges of independence' (Norton, 1965). Whereas the aim of nursing care

| Assessment | | | Medical/social assessment Nursing assessment |
|---|---|---|---|
| | | | **Planning patient care** |
| | | *Remedial* | *Irremedial* |
| | Nursing function | Restoration of self-care abilities | Provision of maximum comfort, happiness and peace of mind; maintenance of optimal level of functioning |
| **Help and assistance** | Skill | Gradual withdrawal of nursing care Teamwork Mental preparation of patients | Maintenance of patient at optimal level of functioning |
| | Goals | Recovery, discharge | Optimal independence, dignity |
| **Optimal independence** | | Home | Performance of activities to optimal level |

**Figure 2**  Concept of geriatric nursing care (Based on Norton et al, 1962; Norton 1965)

for this group must be the giving of maximum comfort, happiness and peace of mind, Norton (1965) warns that nurses must also maintain such patients at their optimal level of functioning. The main components of the geriatric nursing care model are identified in figure 2.

The underlying principle of this model is the nurse's recognition of her primary task as being the provider of nursing care, as opposed to being a facilitator of the medical function. In order to ensure the smooth operation of her caring function, the nurse must be able to work within an organisational system that permits accurate assessment of individual patient's nursing needs, provision of individualised nursing care that is not determined by ward routine, therapeutic use of the ward environment and the provision of total patient care.

Despite the fact that the basic principles of a geriatric nursing care model have been identified from the observations and comments of nurse practitioners in the early 1960s, it is safe to say that the nursing model has lagged greatly behind the development of the geriatric medical care model. In attempting to explain why the geriatric nursing care model has not developed, as evidenced by government and professional reports on the poor standard of nursing care of the hospitalised elderly (Department of Health and Social Security, 1977; Wells, 1980), it is necessary to trace the development of geriatric nursing from the late 1950s and early 1960s to the present. This will be done in the next chapter by a selective survey of geriatric nursing texts and discussion of relevant research studies.

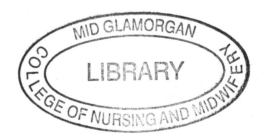

# 2 Geriatric nursing care

The aim of this chapter is to consider the development of geriatric nursing care based on the principles already outlined in chapter 1, which include the need to recognise the primary caring function of the nurse and the need to adopt a positive approach to the health and welfare problems of old people.

The profession's translation of these principles into positive action has also been identified, and comprises such actions as the accurate assessment of each patient's medical, social and nursing care need, the identification of patients' nursing problems and attempting to solve them, the provision of individualised nursing care and the therapeutic use of the ward environment, furniture and equipment (Norton et al, 1962).

It is important at this point to distinguish between the identification of principles of care and the knowledge and skills that a profession develops in order to realise its goals. It would seem that, whereas the medical profession identified the principles of geriatric medical care and proceeded to construct an organisational framework within which to develop specialist knowledge and expertise, the nursing profession has been unable to construct a comparable operational nursing framework around the principles identified by such people as Norton et al (1962) and Rudd (1954). The result has been that, although the geriatric nursing model was identified early on, little real progress has been made in translating such principles into positive action.

The main concern of this chapter, therefore, is to ask why the nursing profession has not applied the principles of the geriatric nursing care model in a more concrete way. In attempting to answer this question, three main areas will be addressed. The first area is a consideration of whether or not the nursing profession accepted the first principle outlined in the geriatric nursing care model, i.e. that the primary function of nursing is basic nursing care, from which all else extends. A further task is to assess the level of knowledge and skill development in geriatric nursing as demonstrated in nursing literature. Finally, the evaluation of the contribution that nursing research has made to the development of geriatric nursing care will be dealt with.

## NURSING'S PRIMARY ORIENTATION – CARE OR CURE?

In explaining the emergence of the geriatric medical model (see figure 1, chapter 1) in the treatment and care of the elderly infirm, it was noted that the principles of the acute medical model – diagnosis, treatment and cure – were applied to the chronic sick sector. However, when one considers the corresponding nursing care model, which could have served as the theoretical framework for the geriatric nursing care model, a major problem arises, namely that nursing does not have an operational model independent of the medical model.

Tiffany (1979, p.3) has described the development of nursing practice as 'a series of stereotyped ritualized acts based upon traditional and imputed preferences which were performed by nurses following the pronouncement of a medical diagnosis'. More recently, Evers (1981a) has argued that the whole basis of nursing in geriatric wards is dominated and controlled by the medical model ethos. She feels that until the medical profession relinquishes its inappropriate claim to the control of long-stay patients and recognises the need to establish a 'caring model' as opposed to a 'curing model', patients will be at risk of depersonalisation and institutionalisation. Evers sees the appropriate model being linked with the provision of care, in which a person-centred philosophy supercedes the traditional disease-oriented model adhered to by the medical profession and acceded to by the nursing profession.

Evers goes on to question the suitability of the nursing profession in taking responsibility for the care of the elderly patients, given its apparent concentration on the disease model and the physical maintenance of the individual, as opposed to the person-centred model advocated by social work practitioners. Miller and Gwynne (1972) and Halliburton and Wright (1974), similarly, have questioned the appropriateness of the nurse to provide care to patients in long-term care settings.

In attempting to explain why geriatric nursing has fallen short of the geriatric care goal, Wells (1980, p.129) identifies the central problem as being that 'nurses do not know why they do what they do'. She continues:

> '[Nurse] training has encouraged nurses to perform ritualistic routines without thinking of the effect of such routines on patient care. Nurses have not been taught how to identify problems in patient care, how to take action to solve such problems, or how to evaluate the effects of nursing action.'

Wells' final comments indicate on whom she lays the blame for the situation in geriatric nursing:

> 'The real constraints to geriatric nursing are neither in the will of the nurse nor the substance of the environment; they exist in the nursing profession's failure to define, describe, teach and facilitate nursing.'

This apparent lack of an operational nursing care model has also been identified by Altschul (1972), who studied the nature of nurse–patient interaction on psychiatric wards. Altschul found it impossible to identify any clear picture of the treatment ideologies that prevailed among nurses or of any theoretical basis upon which nurses entered into interactions with their patients. From this, Altschul (1972, p.192) concluded that 'nurses do not have any identifiable perspective to guide them in their dealings with problematic situations' and that 'there is room for improvement in training to increase the nurse's therapeutic role'.

Towell (1975) also found that, all too often, the nurse's understanding and perspective of her work role was determined by the medical model being used. Studying the behaviour and perceptions of nursing students in three distinctive ward settings within a psychiatric hospital, Towell found that the nurse's reaction to and understanding of patient problems were directly influenced by the prevailing treatment model.

A general conclusion that may be drawn from these observations is that the nursing profession would seem to be guided and manipulated more by external factors (the medical model, social organisation of the ward) than by its own understanding of what constitutes nursing. Although there is an increasing move towards identifying nursing's primary function as the provision of care (Department of Health and Social Security, 1972b; McFarlane, 1976; Henderson, 1980; Griffin, 1983), the profession has been slow to realise the practical implications of such an ideological move.

## Implications of a caring model

McFarlane (1976) has identified the implications for the nursing profession of deciding to follow a nursing model based on care. She shows how care has to be placed within a theoretical framework, which would give meaning and direction to nursing action. First, care provided by the nurse involves a range of nursing activities, from doing everything for the patient, through guiding, supporting and teaching, to being responsible for the environment. The range and focus of the nurse's care is seen to be determined by the individual's health-care needs, which in turn are determined by such factors as age, sex and stage of development. Finally, the nurse's ability to provide meaningful care is influenced by her knowledge and her level of clinical skill development.

Tiffany (1979) further explains the emergence of a nursing model based on the concept of care as comprising the main elements of assessment, help and assistance, and self-care. The nursing assessment is used to determine what level of nursing support is required to meet the individual's normal self-care activities. A second important tool in the nursing care model is the provision of an individualised nursing care plan. Tiffany describes the aim of the care plan as being to offer help and assistance to the individual, according to particular needs that have been identified on a personal level. The nursing care plan is seen as a mechanism that prescribes nursing care, protects the individuality of the patient, promotes independence and permits the nurse to set short- and long-term care goals for her patients.

Thus, the practical application of the nursing model based on the concept of care would appear to be closely linked to the development of individualised patient care and the process of assessing, planning, implementing and evaluating care. It is evident from the comments of Norton et al (1962) that the model of geriatric nursing care that they identified was based on similar modes of action. However, it would appear that the profession has been slow to accept the implication of such a commitment to the concept of care, allowing itself to be directed and controlled by external factors such as the geriatric medical model or a more deeply ingrained custodial care ethos. This may be due to the fact that the profession has not yet achieved full understanding of its caring role and, consequently, has been unable to identify and develop the knowledge and skills needed to realise such professional goals.

## KNOWLEDGE BASE AND SKILL DEVELOPMENT IN GERIATRIC NURSING

In a search of geriatric nursing care articles and texts published between 1962 and 1972, Wells (1980, p.2) found that the state of geriatric nursing knowledge was both vague and diffuse. Whereas the medical diagnosis and treatment of illness in the elderly was adequately covered, Wells noted that it was uncommon to find nursing aspects of patients' problems either clearly discussed or carefully documented. There was no evidence of nursing assessment being undertaken, nor were there guidelines for the planning and implementing of nursing care regimens for patients.

Wells regards geriatric nursing's lack of knowledge and skill development as being symptomatic of its failure to define its area of practice and functions. The development of nursing knowledge and skills is consequently seen to be linked with how nursing solves its theoretical problems. Whereas it may be argued that nursing is now in a better position to define its primary function and to construct the necessary theoretical framework on which to build knowledge and skills, the situation in geriatric nursing practice would still appear to be problematic.

Although the number and range of geriatric nursing publications has increased between 1973 and 1983, the treatment of explicit nursing practice problems, with a few exceptions, remains poor. Pinel (1976) states that, although the nursing journals have readily given space to a number of articles about geriatric nursing, there are very few nurse authors who consistently write articles on this subject.

Clark (1973, p.1452), writing about the nurse's function within the multidisciplinary team, voiced her dissatisfaction with the nurse's skill development:

'In spite of the fact that rehabilitation in the geriatric field has for some years been recognized as a major nursing function, training in remedial and social skills have not been developed to any extent.'

Clark sees the nurses' lack of skill development as having a negative effect on the care they provide:

'Even when nursing staff are wholly conversant with the therapeutic objectives and plan of care, usually they are deficient in the right skills to integrate remedial work into the daily living activities of patients because they have not had an opportunity to develop them.' (p.1453)

A further area that has been identified as being deficient is the lack of individualised nursing care of elderly patients (Reid, 1981). Although the problems identified – lack of clinical nurse experts (Pinel, 1976), lack of therapeutic skills (Clark, 1973) and lack of individualised nursing care – are common to many areas of nursing, a number of factors that exist within geriatric nursing accentuate them. These factors are, briefly, as follows. The first is the still widely held belief that geriatric nursing is just basic nursing care requiring little skill or expertise (Wells, 1980). This notion is reinforced by the use of untrained nursing auxiliary staff in the majority of geriatric wards, particularly in long-stay wards (Hockey, 1976; Baker, 1978; Johnson, 1978). Second, the continued distinction between SEN and SRN grades underlines the dichotomy between acute, technical care and chronic or basic care (Hockey, 1976; Kitson, 1983). Finally, the profession failed to initiate a programme of geriatric nursing experience in the SRN syllabus until 1973 (Reid, 1981).

In a study of the effect of the geriatric module of training on the attitudes of groups of student and pupil nurses, Hooper, (1981a,b) found that many of the negative stereotypes held by the trainees before their ward experience were positively altered by structured programmes of clinical and ward teaching. This would suggest that the relative educational neglect of care of the elderly in the student nurse syllabus may have added to many of the problems now facing nursing practice (Wells, 1980).

The failure of the profession to identify the particular needs of the elderly infirm in a managerially effective way (Rands, 1972) has also affected the development of geriatric knowledge and skills. The principles of patient-centred care advocated by Norton et al (1962) have not been implemented to any great extent in the geriatric ward situation, despite the unprecedented interest displayed by the profession in this approach to care (Grant, 1979). The particular situation of geriatric nursing care serves to underline the profession's lack of clear directives in this area (Rhys Hearn, 1979a,b; Norwich, 1980).

## The development of patient-centred care in geriatric nursing

A growing interest in the organisation of nursing in terms of patient-centred care (Abdellah et al, 1960), together with a series of government reports and studies on the treatment and care of chronic sick and elderly (Robb, 1967; Department of Health and Social Security, 1969, 1971, 1972a; Miller and Gwynne, 1972; Dartington et al, 1974), has helped to focus attention on the individual needs of the hospitalised elderly. Disturbing accounts of institutionalised care and custodial practices have ensured that the nursing profession consider its position as a provider of care.

The central role of the nurse in the provision of individualised care has been described by the British Geriatric Society and Royal College of Nursing (1975) thus:

> 'The quality of the geriatric patient's life in hospital results directly from the standard of care received and is affected not only by *what* happens but also by *how* it happens.'

Joan Kemp (1978, p.198) identifies the dilemma facing nursing when she states:

> 'Basic nurse training prepares the learner for bedside nursing which is physical in plan and short-term in management. This is not adequate preparation for the care of the majority of elderly people in hospital. Those who go into geriatric nursing must develop new skills and adjust to a chair-centred nursing that requires another approach to the patient.'

Despite this recognition of the need for a more patient-centred approach to the delivery of nursing care, few nursing texts reflect the principles and philosophy of individualised care in terms that are translated into positive nursing action on the ward. The majority of texts follow the pattern of presenting a geriatric medical model of care, detailing the development of geriatric units, the concept of progressive patient care and the importance of the multidisciplinary team. The activities of the nurse are variously described, but seldom is her role set out in such a way as to outline the importance of assessing and planning nursing care. Irvine et al (1978), for example, describe the nursing assessment thus:

'One of the questions which the doctor will repeatedly put to the nurse about each patient [is] ... "what can he do" ... this is known as the functional assessment *and it depends on a commonsense way of looking at the patient.*' (p.32, emphasis added)

And again:

'The way the patient should be nursed *may be decided at a glance* but methods have been developed to determine more precisely his nursing needs. (p.33, emphasis added)

Geriatric texts written by medical personnel (Agate, 1979; Chalmers, 1980; Hodkinson, 1981) describe geriatric nursing within a medically oriented model of geriatric care. Hodkinson (1981) warns of the readjustments nurses who were trained in the traditional approach may have to make in caring for the elderly. He adds:

'A policy of helping the patient help himself must replace more custodial attitudes.'

Hodkinson also warns of the nurse's habit of over-protecting the patient, yet nowhere does he consider how the nurse is to acquire a new approach to caring for elderly infirm patients.

For those patients beyond medical reclaim, Hodkinson identifies the nurse as being responsible for creating a total pattern of care that is entirely appropriate to meet the needs of long-stay patients. He describes such a regimen as including opportunities for individual patients to make their own decisions, to enjoy meaningful work and to learn to interact socially. How the nurse is to achieve this is not explained.

Geriatric texts written by nurses (Storrs, 1975; McLeod, 1976) were also found to be vague on the techniques for assessing patient needs and providing individualised care. Furthermore, the main themes identified in nursing journals tended to follow more traditional patterns – descriptions of patients' medical conditions with related nursing care (Sharman, 1972; Brocklehurst, 1973), discussions on the running of the geriatric unit (Dolan et al, 1972; Howell, 1972; Isaacs, 1973; Milligan, 1973; West, 1976) and the multidisciplinary team (Topliss, 1973; McHugh and Chughtai,

1975). A growing interest in the provision of individualised patient care (Grant, 1979), coupled with dissatisfaction with nursing standards in the care of the elderly (Chisholm, 1977; Dent, 1977), has led to a more direct consideration of nurse management regimens on the ward (Cruise, 1978; Mangan, 1982; Skeet, 1982; Storrs, 1982; Watson, 1982).

## The influence of American texts – nursing theories

American texts on geriatric (gerontological) nursing care have also influenced the way in which current knowledge and skills in geriatric nursing are being integrated within the British system. Although the American nursing system is quite distinct from the British system, and comparison between specialties is difficult given the different social and historical backgrounds, one major contribution that American texts of geriatric care have made is in their utilisation of theoretical nursing models by which to identify patient needs and plan care accordingly.

Hogstel (1981, p.22) explains the use of theories of nursing in geriatric care as providing a frame of reference for the individual nurse practitioner through which to 'formulate a model of practice and aid in the evaluation of the outcomes of nursing action'.

She identifies two main theories that are applicable to elderly persons in clinical settings: Orem's self-care theory (Orem, 1980) and Roy's adaptation theory (Riehl and Roy, 1980). Other nursing theories that have been used to describe the dimensions of geriatric nursing care include the psychosocial theory of care utilised by Burnside (1976) and Murray et al (1980), the developmental theory (Yurick et al, 1980) and the coping theory used by Carnevali and Patrick (1979). The psychosocial, developmental and coping theories are adaptations of major psychological and behavioural theories through which nurse practitioners have formulated frameworks for action.

The interpersonal approach to patient care adopted by Burnside (1976) and Murray et al (1980) reflects their orientation toward the psychosocial needs of the elderly. The nurse's role, accordingly, considers such activities as 'one-to-one' relationship therapy with the aged, group therapy and treatment techniques such as reality orientation. Yurick et al (1980) chose to use the major components of developmental theory to define and delineate the parameters of the nurse's function, whereas Carnevali and Patrick (1979) developed a theory of nursing based on the elderly person's ability to cope with and meet his self-care demands. They describe nursing's focus and area of accountability in providing health care as that of helping:

> 'the individual and his family to manage the activities and demands of daily living as these affect and are affected by health and illness, at the same time taking into account the individual's lifestyle.' (p.7)

This definition is similar to the emphasis of Orem's (1980) self-care theory, which states that the nurse should not dictate health-care judgments and practices and impose these on the elderly client. Rather (Hogstel, 1981, p.22):

> 'the nurse through personal knowledge and skill in interviewing and assessing the health care status interprets the data provided by the client and constructs with the client a care plan that is realistic, attainable and measurable from the client's perspective.'

The influence of such approaches on the development of systems of care in Britain can be seen in recent journal articles, e.g. Fleming et al (1983), Watson (1982) and O'Rawe (1982). O'Rawe's description of the care of an elderly gentleman suffering from a variety of medical and social problems, which manifested themselves in a state of self-neglect, is particularly interesting. Using Orem's self-care theory to identify and plan nursing care, O'Rawe provided a system of nursing action that safeguarded the patient's dignity and identified for the nurse the parameters of her caring function, the goal of which was to obtain optimal independence or self-care for the patient. O'Rawe's article marks a trend away from the traditional pattern of viewing geriatric nursing care, demanding from the nurse an independence of action and an ability to provide person-oriented care.

In achieving the goal of optimal independence for the patient, the nurse utilised a theoretical framework based on nursing principles of care rather than on a geriatric medical model. O'Rawe also comments on the expanded role of the nurse within this framework, identifying areas where the nurse would require extra knowledge, training and preparation in order to achieve the best results. A sound theoretical framework, based on the principles of care as the nurse's primary function, and a positive approach to the care of the elderly, operationalised through assessment of individual self-care problems with appropriate nursing action, were identified by O'Rawe as important components in providing nursing care. She further identified the need for the development of more specialised knowledge and skills in dealing with patient problems in this way.

Thus, whereas the geriatric nursing care model (see figure 2 above) identified the principles and the mechanism by which a more positive approach to patient care could be achieved, a selected review of geriatric nursing literature shows a lack of clear development of any of these principles. Interest in the provision of patient-centred care has been impeded by the absence of a clearly defined theoretical framework on which to organise a system of nursing care. Where theoretical frameworks have been used (Burnside 1976; Carnevali and Patrick, 1979; O'Rawe, 1982), they have served to identify and define the parameters of the nurse's function in the care of the elderly, utilising a patient-centred approach to care, which comprises the assessment and planning of nursing care.

## RESEARCH STUDIES

A third area of investigation to be considered in the discussion of why the principles outlined in the geriatric nursing care model were not developed to their full extent is a selected review of research studies that have focused upon the care of the institutionalised elderly. The review is confined to British studies dealing with the care of the elderly, the studies being divided into three main methodological categories. These are 'descriptive', 'workload/patient dependency' and 'social systems' approaches. Particular attention will be paid to how the methodological framework influenced the formulation of the results and conclusions arrive at in each study.

### Descriptive studies

The two main studies included in this section are those of Norton et al (1962) and Wells (1980). The investigation by Norton et al concentrated on studying the basic nursing care of old people in hospital, describing its constraints and then attempting to show how such problems might arise. Norton also claimed that it was as much her goal to identify the problems facing geriatric nursing as it was to suggest possible solutions. Problem identification is seen as an important component in descriptive studies.

Sister Mary Xavier, commenting in the epilogue of the report, summarised the guiding principles that dictate the methodological framework of the study:

'Throughout all sections of this report, the treatment of patients as individuals has emerged as a prominent factor.'

A concern to provide patient-centred care determined the study framework; a 24-hour analysis of 18 patients' nursing needs was undertaken by the researchers, using continuous, non-participant observation techniques. From this analysis, the quantity and quality of nursing care was assessed in relation to each patient's basic nursing needs. External variables were considered in terms of a descriptive account of the suitability of ward furniture, equipment and patient clothing.

One of the main conclusions reached by Norton et al was the need to assess patient's individual nursing needs and to draw up ways of meeting these needs without the constraints of the ward routines. They advocated the use of individual nursing care plans, together with more therapeutic and knowledgeable use of the environment – furniture, equipment and clothing.

Wells (1980) similarly considered a range of possible factors that may have influenced the type of nursing care provided for the hospitalised elderly. Again, basing her methodological framework on the principle of individualised patient care, Wells investigated the effect both of external factors (environment, ward equipment and furniture, ancillary services) and internal factors (nurses' attitudes toward the elderly, their knowledge of geriatric nursing problems, management constraints) on the nurses' ability to give personalised care. Data were collected in a variety of ways, using information-gathering tools that would provide optimal amounts of reliable observations – check-lists, questionnaires, patient dependency scales and non-participant observational methods.

The climax of Wells' investigation came in a study of nurse–patient communication, the majority of cases of which she described as being related to procedures or tasks and not focused on the patient. Wells chose to view nurse–patient verbal communication as a visible sign of the nurse–patient relationship, which she concluded was 'limited and not very meaningful' (Wells, 1980, p.123).

Wells attributes the lack of individualised patient care, as exemplified by poor nurse–patient verbal communication, to the nurses' failure to focus their ward work on the specific needs of individual patients and their failure to provide nursing records of patient preferences. Despite identifying and considering several external factors that might have influenced the way the nurse cared for her patient, Wells concludes her study by stating that geriatric nursing's failure to provide adequate nursing care is the major responsibility of the nursing profession. She advocates the development of a grade of nurse to act as a 'change agent' to improve the situation and the quality of care, thus ensuring a more patient-centred approach to the care of the elderly.

Both studies serve the useful purpose of describing geriatric nursing. It is important to remember that any interpretation of the observed situation is based on a comparison of the observed situation with a preferred or ideal situation. In both studies, the ideal situation is that of patient-focused care, as it relates primarily to the provision of individual self-care needs.

## Workload/patient dependency studies

The majority of British studies have tended to focus on particular tasks involved in geriatric nursing work and the impact on these tasks of the characteristics of the patients, rather than attempt to describe the constraints of geriatric nursing care. Such workload/patient dependency studies are based on the primary assumption that nursing can be regarded as a series of activities that can be defined, observed and counted, the nature and duration of which can be calculated according to the patient's dependency level. With knowledge of such information, the staffing levels required to deliver care to groups of patients with different dependency needs can be calculated. A further assumption on which this approach is based is that the nursing care a patient requires is observable, finite, measurable and relatively stable when it has been prescribed, and that there is an optimum length of time to carry out certain activities according to different dependency categories (Redfern, 1981).

Major contributions in this area include studies by Goddard

(1953, 1963), Adams and McIlwraith (1963), Scottish Home and Health Department (1967), Callaghan (1968) and, more recently, the series of investigations undertaken by Rhys Hearn and colleagues (Rhys Hearn and Potts, 1978; Rhys Hearn, 1979a,b; Rhys Hearn and Howard, 1980). With the exception of Rhys Hearn's work, the majority of studies discuss the nurses' activities carried out in geriatric wards in terms of the proportion of time spent on various tasks, those related directly to the patient being classed as either 'basic' or 'technical' tasks.

The main drawback of these studies is that the workload is based on the *observed* practices on the ward rather than on the *prescribed* or *ideal* levels of care. Furthermore, consideration of individual patient needs is impossible given the fact that patients are usually grouped into between three and five major care categories, from which average times for care are deduced. Rhys Hearn's series of investigations, however, has attempted to provide more individualised care by using nursing information from each patient's care plan in order to predict the overall nursing workload of the ward (Wade and Snaith, 1981). This method is particularly attractive on two counts: first, it utilises the most specific set of nursing data for each ward patient, and, second, it takes into consideration rather more intangible nursing activities such as providing support, supervising patients and help with rehabilitation.

Reporting on a trial of this 'package', in which nursing staff were allocated in accordance with the nurse's identification of the patients' optimal nursing requirements, Rhys Hearn (1979b) noted that 'in no case was the care given equivalent to the care prescribed'.

Thus, despite the presence of optimal numbers of nurses and the existence of individualised nursing care plans, Rhys Hearn found that nurses were still unable to adjust their routines to incorporate such activities as emotional support and rehabilitation procedures. Norwich (1980) similarly reported that nursing staff tended to spend extra nursing time in physical care activities rather than in providing psychosocial or therapeutic support. Savage et al (1979) also recorded similar nursing behaviour in psychogeriatric wards.

It would appear that the provision of adequate staffing levels does not automatically ensure an increase in the range of activities performed by nurses or in the meeting of patients' prescribed needs. In considering workload studies, Baker (1978, p.31, emphasis added) comments:

> 'The question of efficient and effective nursing cannot just be dealt with by a mechanical appraisal of the allocation of resources in the course of carrying out a particular task. The question arises as to *what are the ramifications of the task.*'

Although attractive as a quantitative methodological tool and as a management tool, studies on workload and patient dependency will not be able to solve the problem of why nurses do not or cannot meet the prescribed needs of patients in the ideal staffing situation (Rhys Hearn, 1979a,b; Savage et al, 1979). Knowledge of this fact, however, enables one to consider other factors that may affect the nurse's ability to provide more patient-focused care.

## Social systems studies

The final group of research studies to be considered have based analyses of their observations on a 'social systems' framework rather than a workload or descriptive approach. The distinguishing characteristics of the social systems approach have been described by Towell (1979) as comprising three main elements. These are: the social action perspective (Silverman, 1970; Eldridge, 1971) – the way in which various participants in health-care settings themselves define the situation in which they are involved and what purposes and norms guide their actions; the setting/arena (Strauss et al, 1963) – that is, the setting in which different professional, non-professional and client groups meet, each with their own perspectives and purposes, to work out, through negotiation, the courses of action that add up to more or less enduring patterns of work and forms of organisation; and a consideration of structural conditions – this refers to the division of labour, the distribution of power between groups involved and the technical and personal resources available for the tasks in question.

Four main research studies have been identified that use this analytical framework to explain the nursing care given to hospitalised elderly patients. These are studies by Towell (1975), Dartington et al (1974), Baker (1978) and Evers (1981a,b, 1982a,b).

Although Towell's research was based on psychiatric patient care, he included in his analysis the nursing care of psychogeriatric patients. Through participant observation techniques Towell attempted to build up a detailed picture of everyday life in hospital and to identify the meanings that nurses gave to their work and their relationships with patients in various settings. Towell found that, very often, the meaning that nurses conferred upon particular nursing care situations was determined by their interpretation of the ideologies of treatment of the ward and the patterns of ward organisation. Thus, on the admission ward, where the medical model of care was used, Towell noted that nurses gave meaning to the actions of patients through interpretations based on the 'medical model'. There the nurses used the diagnostic categories and medical symptoms of patients as an indicator of the level of nursing care and attention required. The nurses' experience on the geriatric wards, however, was influenced more by the need for the completion of rigidly scheduled routines based on the physical needs of the patients than by any medical goal (Towell, 1975, p.141).

Towell concludes that the lack of development of the nurse's therapeutic role is due to the dominant medical model, which exerts a strong influence on the definition of tasks and the allocation of resources. He also blames the formal organisation of the hospital, with its parallel nursing and medical hierarchies, and the traditional centralisation of control as contributory factors in constraining the ward-based development of new nursing treatment ideologies.

Using a similar analytical framework, Dartington et al (1974) studied the level of stress experienced by nurses in geriatric hospitals that advocated a progressive patient care policy. The researchers specifically looked at the settings in which the range of professional and non-professionals met to negotiate the course of action or treatment regimens for groups of elderly people. The study also looked at the relationship that existed between the geriatric hospital and the community, and found that whereas the hospital was overtly there to provide treatment that the ideology of progressive patient care emphasised, it was also being asked by society to take responsibility for old people. Thus, Dartington et al found that not only were staff dealing with ambivalent social attitudes to the care they were providing but that they were also faced with the conflict between pushing patients to be independent, as advocated in the philosophy of progressive patient care, and wanting to provide patients with a level of care likely to encourage continuing dependence. The resultant stress experienced by nursing staff was seen to be a feature of opposing social and medical orientations, together with the absence of a clearly defined theoretical framework within which to interpret the nurse's legitimate nursing function.

Baker's (1978) study addressed itself chiefly to the question of how nurses looking after the elderly perceived their patients and their job, as revealed by what they said and did. In attempting to explain how nurses came to define their patients, Baker identified prevalent societal attitudes to the elderly, referring to their diminished social status (de Beauvoir, 1973), and the tendency of society to isolate them. The wider values of society were seen to be reinforced in the structural conditions in the geriatric ward situation. Here, Baker observed that the division of labour and distribution of power was such that work was valued according to its conformity to the medical model of treatment and cure. Thus, at the top of the 'pecking order' was the assessment ward, where patients achieved the cure goal and, in consequence, escaped the worst aspects of the geriatric label. (Baker found that nurses in assessment wards tended not to view patients as totally dependent, socially diminished and unreliable, as was the case in the other wards, particularly the long-stay ones.) Baker also reported that the orientation of nursing staff in long-stay wards was toward the completion of ward routines, which were described as 'barely adequate to meet patients' minimal needs for assistance with activities of daily living.'

The existence and toleration of such a regimen of care – termed 'routine geriatric style of nursing' – was seen as a direct reflection of the way in which the attributes of geriatric patients were perceived by nurses at ward level and above. Nurses' perspectives were thought to be moulded by the medical model of geriatric care, which conferred greater importance on remediable than long-term care patients. The setting in which geriatric nursing care took place was seen by Baker to be a significant factor in the acceptance of the routine geriatric style of nursing, both in terms of location and the managerial system that developed between nurses on the ward and the nursing hierarchy, and of the relations between the medical consultants and nursing hierarchy.

Although Baker argues that, in order to explain the unsatisfactory condition of geriatric care, consideration must be given to a number of 'interlocking and mutually reinforcing factors' (Baker, 1978, p.295), she concludes that, in order radically to alter the situation, attention must be focused on 'the perceptions and morale of those who have to implement ... policies of ward level i.e. the ward nurses'. Thus, despite the wider social systems analysis that characterized Baker's approach, her belief is that the success of any reform in the organisation and delivery of care depends on the perception and morale of the nursing staff. To this end, she suggests action aimed at improving nursing education and effecting ways of 'sensitizing the profession to the shortcomings, the challenge and the nursing potential surrounding the care of dependent elderly'.

Commenting on Baker's analysis of the social structure of geriatric nursing and her subsequent call on the nursing profession to initiate solutions, Evers (1982a,b) feels that such conclusions are unrealistic. She questions how nurses are to solve, alone, a set of nursing practice and management problems derived from a multiplicity of interlocking factors far beyond the direct control of the nurse. Evers argues that it is only by looking at the nature of social relationships that exist within an organisational structure in terms of how they affect the patient that adequate solutions may be obtained.

By considering the nature of the long-stay care task in hospital, Evers' (1981a) intention was to discover how, in an institutional setting, a caring environment could be created in which some level of quality of life was guaranteed. She also attempted to explore possible ways of changing the organisation of such a task with a view to achieving maximum positive care outcomes for patients. In looking at the practice of geriatrics in relation to the treatment policies outlined in government documents (Department of Health and Social Security, 1977, 1978) and, in particular, by contrasting the approach to remedial and long-stay patients, Evers found that, by focusing on the patient's experience, she was able to determine whether the outcomes were positive for both patient and staff. For the remedial patients Evers found that their career pattern accrued to medical model objectives, whereas for long-stay patients attempts to meet such objectives were not apparent, resulting in a routinised type of care.

Through analysis of the career patterns of long-stay patients, Evers felt it was possible to identify conditions under which more patient-centred care might be fulfilled. She also felt that the provision of such care – which she termed tender loving care –

was closely linked to the social relationships among all the participants in ward work and, in particular, to the relationship between the consultant and the ward sister. As a result of concentrating on the personal experiences of long-stay patients in eight different ward settings and of utilising a participant observation technique, Evers identified two dominant modes of nursing care treatment – personalised warehousing (characterised by increased personal choice, increased social interaction, increased chance of leaving the ward for diversional activities for long-stay patients) and minimal warehousing (minimal personal choice, social isolation, the ward seen as a closed environment for long-stay patients). Evers then identified a range of organisational factors that she considered to be responsible for determining which model prevailed. She concluded (Evers, 1981a, p.62):

> 'It appeared that the crucial difference between personalized and minimal warehousing wards concerned the ward sister's scheduling strategy and interrelated with this the structure of social relations among the members of the multidisciplinary team; most importantly between ward sisters and consultant geriatricians.'

Evers argues that when the nurse is given responsibility for the long-stay care of patients, the care becomes more personalised, whereas if the medical profession fails to recognise the central role of the nurse, the patient is more likely to experience depersonalised care. By conferring legal, administrative and professional authority on the nursing profession for the care of long-stay patients, Evers suggests that conditions are created whereby the care task, being organisationally segregated from the medically dominated cure model, can be seen as valid, important and legitimate work to be performed within the health-care system. One cautionary note must be that merely freeing the nursing profession from the domination of the medical model does not automatically mean that it is able to provide person-centred care. Like Baker, Evers recommends the development of a special training programme, together with the creation of an organisational infrastructure that would value and support the performance of long-term care tasks by accountable and skilled nurse professionals.

## Discussion of research findings

Perhaps one of the most important factors highlighted in the research studies is an indication of the complexity of the problems confronting the nursing profession in trying to find solutions to the care of the hospitalised elderly. The interaction of factors has been clearly demonstrated in the 'social system' studies (Dartington et al, 1974; Towell, 1975; Baker, 1978; Evers, 1981a, 1982a,b), in which the domination of the medical model has tended to be blamed for many of the observed shortcomings. The domination of the medical model is thought to be due to the orientation of the health-care organisational structure and the management system, which are geared to work toward the cure goal in preference to the goal of care.

When the medical model varied in form (Towell, 1975), the orientation and experiences of the nursing profession were also affected. This observation would tend to suggest that the nursing profession does not have a complementary model by which to organise its caring activities. However, both Baker (1978) and Evers (1981a) identified groups of nursing staff who provided a level of care that was more personalised and tended not to conform to the standard routinised style of care. Neither researcher could identify external factors such as environment, quality of furniture and equipment, dependency level and age of patient, etc. as being responsible for the change in the pattern of care.

Evers felt that the explanation for the two styles of care (which she termed personalised warehousing and minimal warehousing) was directly linked to the relationship between the ward sister and the consultant geriatrician. Baker (1978), however, adopted a different analysis in explaining the difference between the majority of nurses who gave 'routine geriatric care' and the minority who were found to provide 'non-routine' or 'personalised' geriatric care. Baker tended to think that the main reason for the different approaches lay more in the personal development and the professional beliefs and attitudes of the individual nurse than in the social relationship between the nurse and the medical practitioner.

Baker's analysis may be given some credibility by the conclusions of Rhys Hearn (1979a,b) and Norwich (1980) on the nurses' ability to provide optimal care. When strict structural and organisational constraints, such as lack of staff and lack of time to provide patient-centred care, were controlled, nurses were still unable to provide patients with the ideal care that they themselves had prescribed. These observations indicate a more serious problem within the nurse's own perception and understanding of her nursing function.

Wells' (1980) comments similarly reflect her conviction that the problems confronting geriatric nursing care are primarily based on the profession's failure to define, prescribe and teach nursing rather than on external factors, although, as the research studies have shown, external factors have a marked influence. It may be that the influence of the medical model, as described by Evers, has seemed dominant because the nursing profession has still to identify its own particular orientation.

The research studies have, therefore, attested to the impression that the geriatric nursing care model has not been developed to any significant degree in the majority of geriatric care settings observed. The predominating type of care provided by nursing staff is best described as routinised. Whereas a minority of nurses were found to provide more personalised care, no clear explanation was given for this. One interpretation was based on the social relationship between the ward sister and the medical personnel, the medical profession giving up its responsibility for the care of the long-stay patients and confering it upon the nursing profession. An alternative analysis preferred to explain the phenomenon as being linked with the professional ideology and standards of the individual nurse and the subsequent translation of these ideals into more positive care of the elderly.

Thus, in terms of the two main principles of the geriatric care model – the recognition of the nurse's primary caring function and the adoption of a positive approach to the health and welfare problems of old people – it is evident that the nursing profession has failed to confront the complex managerial and organisational problems involved in providing patient-centred care. The nursing profession has only recently begun to agree on the need to recognise and define its actions in terms of patients' basic self-care needs (McFarlane, 1976), and, similarly, developments toward ensuring the provision and execution of individualised nursing care have been a recent priority (Grant, 1979).

Nursing literature needs to reflect the nursing care model more clearly, and, particularly, it needs to identify the range of skills required by the nurse working with the elderly infirm. Above all, it would seem that geriatric nursing care requires a theoretical framework on which to build the dimensions of its caring function. It is to the theoretical framework for geriatric nursing care that we now turn.

# 3 Geriatric nursing framework

Before the range of complex structural, organisational and ideological problems facing geriatric nursing can begin to be solved, the profession needs to develop a theoretical framework that provides boundaries and sets guidelines to explain the nurse's function in geriatric care. The aim of this chapter, therefore, is to identify the essential components of a possible theoretical framework, to demonstrate how this framework can provide structure, direction and meaning to geriatric nursing care and; finally, to explain how the framework may be used as an important feature in the methodological approach to this research study of the nursing care of the hospitalised elderly in Northern Ireland.

The theoretical framework, based on Orem's (1980) self-care theory, will be contrasted with the geriatric nursing care model identified by Norton et al (1962). Although there are certain features similar to both frameworks, the more detailed self-care theoretical framework based on Orem's approach is favoured to that of Norton et al.

## NURSING THEORY – PROBLEM IDENTIFICATION

It would appear that the question most often asked about nursing theory is not whether it exists but, more interestingly, whether it contributes anything of value to the practice situation (Hardy, 1974; Stevens, 1979; Johnson, 1983). The position taken in this discussion is one of accepting the existence of nursing theory and, from this basis, arguing for the need to identify and develop the nursing theory most appropriate to the geriatric nursing care situation.

Dickoff and James (1968) see nursing theory's aim as acting as a guide, control or shaper of reality but not being, in itself, 'reality'. A nursing theory attempts to describe or explain the phenomenon called nursing (Stevens, 1979, quoted by Johnson, 1983). McFarlane (1980) describes theory as consisting of a pattern of logical constructs into which all facts relevant to a phenomenon can be fitted. Theory not only provides a framework on which to organise facts but, according to McFarlane, also provides a means whereby relationships can be specified, thus permitting understanding, prediction and the exercise of influence and control (McFarlane, after Kerlinger, 1973).

Smith (1982) further describes theories as 'abstractions which may be translated into action through models.' She explains the link between theory and models as:

> 'models being lower representations of theory located in reality ... A model, as a reflection of theory, may be subject to empirical study which validates or disproves the theory or causes revision in a theory's formulation.' (p.117)

This emphasis on the need for nursing theory to be linked to the practice situation is a notion held by Dickoff et al (1968, p.415), who claim:

> 'theory is born in practice, refined in research and returns to practice.'

In considering the origin of theory, they link an individual's ability to observe and criticise a situation with the first steps towards problem identification and analysis. They describe a problem as:

> 'a sophistication of criticism to the point of being articulate about *what* is at fault along with *a desire* to remove the fault ... A problem is a director of inquiry – having a problem – rather than a mere worry, criticism or vague discontent – is having both impetus (interest and energy) and direction (initial conceptualisation) for using thought to remove the fault identified by the problem.'

They continue:

> 'This move from discomfort felt in practice to articulation of the difficulty and thence to first speculative and then eventual practical resolution of the difficulty epitomizes that theory is born in practice and must return to practice.'

Norton et al's (1962) study is a good example of how the identification of practical nursing problems may lead to the development of a more theoretical perspective on nursing problems. Discontentment with nursing practice led the researchers to identify specific nursing care problems. Norton (1967, 1970), Norton et al (1962) and Wells (1980) have commented on the complex nature of the nursing problems, Wells further noting the apparent lack of conceptualisation of many of the problems by geriatric nursing staff (Wells, 1980, p.130). She did find, however, that nurses were able to criticise the situation, but such criticisms were described in terms of worries and discontent rather than being an 'articulation of what is at fault along with a desire to remove the fault' (Dickoff et al, 1968, p.418).

This differentiation between the nurse's ability to criticise on the one hand and identify problems on the other was thought to be an important concept in the understanding and analysis of the nurse's role in the care of the elderly. Dickoff et al (1968) do not explain how the individual moves from the 'criticism' stage to the 'problem identification' stage, the latter characterising the commencement of the analytical approach to nursing practice. A possible explanation of what characterises those individuals who identify and solve problems, as compared with those who criticise, may be linked with what Dickoff and James (1968) have called the influence of 'professional purpose'.

## A theoretical framework for a practice discipline

Dickoff and James (1968) argue that the type of theoretical framework needed for a professional discipline is characterised by three main features: namely, it is *action-oriented*; that the professional shapes reality as opposed to being a 'doer who merely tends the cogs of reality according to prescribed patterns'; and that the professional shapes reality according to an articulated purpose and in the light of reality. The authors summarize by stating (Dickoff and James, 1968, p.199, emphasis added):

> 'a theory for a profession or practice discipline must provide for more than mere understanding or "describing" or even predicting reality and must *provide conceptualization specially intended to guide the shaping of reality to that professional's professional purpose.'*

Hence it may be that the difference between nurses who 'criticise' and nurses who 'identify problems' rests with their conceptual-isations about their nursing function, which consequently guides the focus of their professional action. Dickoff and James (1968) go on to argue that if nursing is a profession, *it must have a theoretical framework, which aims to shape reality based on a conception of nursing goals, and articulated methods by which to achieve those goals*. In order to reach such goals, nursing theory must be seen at a level capable of guiding action to the production of 'prescribed reality', i.e. reality that has been prescribed by professional perspectives and standards. Theory at this level is described by them as situation producing theory, where the three essential components are goal content, prescription for activity and survey list.

The main structures of the theory are goal content and prescription. Goal content is described as the conceptualisation of an objective of nursing care, through which positive outcomes will be achieved. Dickoff et al (1968, p.424) warn against the danger of having as goals 'shadowy high ideals' that are impossible to convert into practice reality. They state:

> 'the theory must render articulate the conception of the kinds of situations that are to be brought into existence as widespreadly as possible.'

Prescriptions can be viewed as models of action that aim to achieve the goals outlined by the theoretical and professional perspective of those involved in the activity (Dickoff et al, 1968). They have three important characteristics: prescriptions are commands, they give directions; they are characterised by action geared toward a specified end; and they are commands directed to some specified agent.

The third element of the theoretical framework of a practice discipline is the survey list. The survey list serves as a reminder of the range of variables that can affect both the goal content and the prescription. Included in the survey list are such items as: the individual or thing performing the activity (the *agent*); the recipient of the activity (termed *patiency*); the context in which the activity is performed, which may be environmental or structural constraints (the *framework*); the identifiable end-point of the activity where the nurse's actions are no longer required (the *terminus*); the organisational framework (the *procedure*); and, finally, the *dynamics* of the situation – the determination of the energy source of the activity.

In an effort to elucidate the theoretical framework outlined above and to demonstrate how it may be used both in an explanatory and predictive capacity in geriatric nursing care, one of Wells' (1980) investigations will be analysed using this framework. The particular study involved an assessment of the methods used to provide hospitalised patients with personalised clothing. The objective or goal content of such a scheme was to ensure patient dignity and self-respect through the provision of personalised clothing. Such goals were advocated both by professionals (Irvine et al, 1978; Hodkinson, 1981) and by government recommendation (Department of Health and Social Security, 1972b). The implications of such a change in policy were identified early on by Trott (1970), the first clothing manager, who listed some of the main difficulties – selection, issue, sorting, clothing, marking, storage, repairs and laundering.

When Wells came to assess the operation of the personalised clothing system on the ward, she found that it was informal and unplanned. The design of clothes was poor, the supply unpredictable, no-one had overall responsibility for clothing and 'no-one had the time to completely work out their own problems in each area'. Thus, in terms of the goal content, although the staff agreed in principle with the provision of personalised clothing, Wells found that they had no clear conceptualisation of the process of action by which such a goal could be realised. Prescriptions for action were vague and unformulated, while, at ward level, the agent responsible for the performance of the task was restricted on all sides: as the performer or agent of the task, the nurse was constrained by a variety of more clearly articulated priorities, e.g. getting patients washed, fed and toiletted. Wells also notes that nowhere did the nurse receive education in dressing techniques and that the organisational structure or framework within which the nurse operated was unco-ordinated, no-one taking responsibility for the provision, delivery, maintenance and assessment of the scheme.

Neither the way in which the system was organised nor the motivation and direction of those involved seemed to be able to achieve the stated goal, i.e. the elderly patient's dignity and self-respect being upheld through the provision of well-fitting, suitable day clothing. It would appear, therefore, according to Wells' own analysis and through interpretation with the theoretical framework, that failure to achieve the stated goal was linked to the lack of detailed prescription of the steps involved in goal realisation. Wells herself suggests five steps toward ensuring goal content (1980, pp.50–61). These are: assessing the operational policies of departments involved in the process; ensuring a common understanding of the goal content; developing a plan of action; establishing effective channels of communication; and appointing a specific agent/worker to monitor activity.

Thus, the elements of this theoretical framework can be used both to describe activity and to identify possible areas of change. A central feature of the framework is the specification of the goal content, as this determines the nature of the prescriptions for activity. The goals of action may be specific, as in the example of the goal to provide a personalised clothing service to geriatric patients, or they may be more general, e.g. the nursing goal of action may be identified as the provision of assistance to those in need of basic self-care (Henderson, 1966; Orem, 1980), to help the individual to adapt to changes in his health status (Roy, 1980) or to help the individual to achieve health (King, 1981; Clark, 1982). The choice of goal content will obviously affect the range and orientation of nursing action needed to meet the goal. The most appropriate goal content for geriatric nursing care will be considered next.

## CONCEPTS BASIC TO GERIATRIC NURSING CARE

### The right to choose

The main elements of a framework defining the nurse's function in geriatric nursing care include the provision of dignity and self-esteem (British Geriatric Society and Royal College of Nursing, 1975) and optimal independence (Department of Health and Social Security, 1977). Achieving and maintaining one's optimal level of independence has been increasingly linked with the elderly person's right to control his situation and to choose a particular type of assistance (Norman, 1980; Hobman, 1982). The right to choose also involves a certain measure of 'risk-taking', a feature that is increasingly seen as an integral part of life and which is linked with the individual's right to self-determination.

## Self-care

Another concept that has particular significance is that of 'self-care'. Levin et al (1979) define self-care as:

> 'a process whereby a lay person functions on his/her own behalf in health promotion and prevention and in disease detection and treatment.'

Williamson and Danaher (1978) identify the following four roles for self-care: health maintenance and disease prevention, self diagnosis, medication and treatment, and patient participation in the health-care services. They also acknowledge the fact that the majority of individuals provide their own health care when faced with illness, and suggest that the role of the professional health worker ought to be one of consultation, detection and prevention rather than of being 'healers' or 'health providers'. Hobman (1982) similarly argues that given the changing trends in illness and in the population profile – more chronic illness coupled with an increasingly aged population – individuals must be made aware of their own responsibility in providing self-care. This would involve such factors as a healthy life-style, diet, a well adapted environment and a network support for particular situations.

This emphasis on self-care, with its increase in responsibility for the individual to provide for and maintain himself at his optimal level of health, has implications for the nurse's perception of her caring role. A central premise of this thesis is that the nurse's primary function is to provide care to those individuals unable to meet their basic self-care needs. Thus, when the nurse is faced with an individual unable to provide adequate self-care, her task comprises meeting his immediate needs and helping him to reach a stage where he can once again meet his own self-care needs. The nurse, therefore, does not 'take over' but, by consulting with the patient and permitting him to progress towards his optimal level of self-care, guarantees the patient's sense of dignity and self-respect as well as permitting a measure of risk-taking and choice-making.

## A PROPOSED THEORETICAL FRAMEWORK FOR GERIATRIC NURSING CARE

The concept of self-care was chosen as the most appropriate vehicle on which to build a framework for geriatric nursing care. The self-care theory for nursing advanced by Orem (1971) and the Nursing Development Conference Group (1973) has been widely used in the practice setting, particularly in America (Backscheider, 1974; Joseph, 1980; Riehl and Roy, 1980). Although its use in the geriatric ward situation has not been as widely documented, there are a few exceptions (Hogstel, 1981; O'Rawe 1982). This lack of theory utilisation was thought to be due more to a general disinterest in care of the elderly than to the inappropriateness of the self-care theory framework. With this in mind, Orem's self-care theory for nursing has been adopted as the proposed theoretical framework for geriatric nursing care.

Self-care, the basic concept of Orem's theory has been described by Joseph (1980) as being founded on six premises. The first is that self-care is based on voluntary actions; the second, that it is based on deliberate and thoughtful judgment that leads to appropriate action in which the individual becomes the principal agent in guiding, directing and regulating his behaviour. Third, self-care is a requirement of every person and is a universal requisite for meeting human needs, and, when care is not maintained, a detrimental change in health occurs. Fourth, adults have rights and responsibilities to care for themselves, aware that developmental and health-related factors affect their ability to perform the activity. The final two premises state that self-care is behaviour which evolves through a combination of social and cognitive experiences and is learned through one's interpersonal relations, communication and culture, and that self-care contributes to the self-esteem and self-image of a person and is directly affected by self-concept.

Self-care, therefore, is viewed as a function necessary for the maintenance of life and healthy living. In situations where the individual is unable to provide a level of self-care that will ensure health, it is the nurse's responsibility to provide the necessary assistance and support. Nursing assistance may arise from the individual experiencing an inability to meet a particular self-care need due to his stage of development, his state of health or a disturbance in one of his basic self-care patterns. Orem (1980) calls these situations developmental, health deviational and universal self-care requirements.

Universal self-care requirements are basic human needs that are constantly present and must be met in order to maintain a healthy state. They include the maintenance of adequate nutrition, hydration, oxygenation, elimination, psychological and social needs of individuals, the need for activity and rest, protection from hazards and the need for 'normalcy' – the opportunity to live out as normal a life-style as possible. Nursing's involvement with the individual's developmental and health requirements is introduced when features of universal self-care activities have been altered by such developmental changes as pregnancy and old age or by pathological change, all of which create problems for the individual in successfully meeting self-care requirements. The nurse's responsibility in such situations is to provide means by which the individual will be able to cope with the new self-care demands made on him.

When an individual requires help to meet his self-care needs, the nurse has a legitimate responsibility to initiate modes of action with a view to helping him meet those needs. How she recognises, interprets and meets the self-care needs of the patient depends on her ability to prescribe a series of nursing activities that are directly guided by the goal content, the aim of the nursing activity. In Orem's theoretical framework, the goal has been identified as 'optimal self-care' in which nursing action strives to maintain the individual at his optimal level of self-care and independence.

The prescription or sequences of activities identified to realise the goal content have also been clearly identified by Orem (1980). Characteristics of the patient to be taken into consideration are those involved in his basic ability to initiate and perform health activities for himself in order to maintain life, health and well-being. This is termed his 'self-care agency' and will be affected by his knowledge, skill, habits, developmental stage and motivation. When the individual's ability to provide self-care falls below a certain minimum level that is considered necessary to sustain 'healthful' living, he is said to have a 'self-care deficit'. The nurse's response to this situation is to identify those activities needing to be performed by the individual or assisted by the nurse in order to accomplish therapeutic self-care. Orem has identified a variety of methods of nursing assistance to help meet patients' therapeutic self-care needs. These include acting for or doing for another, guiding another, supporting another, providing an environment that promotes personal development and teaching another.

Determination of the type of nursing assistance needed by each patient is based on an assessment of the patient's therapeutic 'self-care demand'. Three main nursing systems have been identified, which reflect the needs of the patient and the most appropriate helping method required of the nurse (Joseph, 1980, p.138):

1.  *Wholly compensatory system:* In this system the patient does not have the resources to meet his therapeutic self-care needs and, consequently, the accomplishment of all self-care activities becomes the responsibility of the nurse. The method of nursing assistance that is most appropriate in this case is that of acting and doing for.

2.  *Partially compensatory system:* Both the patient and the nurse are able to perform therapeutic self-care measures within this system. The nurse may use all five methods of helping, ranging from providing total assistance to encouraging and teaching the patient how to perform an activity.

3.  *Supportive – educative system:* Here the patient has the resources to meet his demands but may need nursing assistance in such areas as decision-making, behaviour control, acquisition of knowledge or skill or recovery of self-confidence and self-esteem. In this system, the patient is able to perform, or can perform, required measures of self-care, but cannot do so without assistance.

The prescription phase also requires a nursing system that collects relevant information about the patient's self-care requirements, assesses the most appropriate mode of nursing action and plans particular methods of assistance. The characteristics of this system will be influenced by the nurse's judgment of the situation and by her ability to construct appropriate methods of assistance within the organisational and structural constraints of the ward. The range of factors that may influence the prescribed action of the nurse working toward the goal of optimal self-care can be outlined in terms of the survey list (Dickoff and James, 1968).

The relative efficiency of the nurse as an agent in the process will depend on her ability to evaluate the patient's therapeutic self-care demand. The extent of her nursing assistance will also depend on her level of knowledge and skill development and her ability to design and control the situation. Characteristics of the patient – including age, developmental stage, sex, health state, family support and motivational and knowledge factors – will determine the extent to which he will be able to regain control of his self-care or require continued support from the nurse.

Both the organisational framework and the design and planning of a system of nursing care will affect the goal. A framework that is flexible and accommodates the variation in patients' self-care needs must provide effective communication channels between the individuals involved in providing and receiving care. It further requires a minimum standard of environmental factors that may be used to enhance patient independence and well-being.

Finally, the survey list takes account of the dynamics of the activity, and, according to McFarlane (1980), both the nurse and the patient have an effect on this. The nurse's knowledge and skills influence the design, initiation and control of the system, whereas the patient's characteristics influence the effectiveness of the activity. The nurse also affects the situation by the strength of her motivation and the goals that drive her to provide a particular type of care (Dickoff et al, 1968). The latter authors go on to state:

> 'The goals under which people work or live themselves constitute factors which must be taken account of in activity since these goals have ramifications, both positive and negative, for the activity.' (p.431)

Such goals, which may provide impetus and direction for the performance of a professional activity, include service motivation and the desire to help, to perform a task competently and to experience a feeling of self-fulfilment in having performed a task to one's optimum ability.

Dickoff et al see these factors as having quite a significant influence on the way nursing is performed. Such features may inculcate, sustain and increase service motivation, whereas other factors such as frustration may decrease or inhibit service motivation. The link between service motivation and the competent performance of tasks is a close one, one's feeling of self-fulfilment being related to the capacity to conceptualise both the overall role and the particular activity, thus giving meaning to each task performed. In other words, the successful outworking of the nurse's caring function is seen by the authors to be intimately linked to her perception of her own motivation and orientations in conjunction with her knowledge and skills. Similarly, Orem's self-care framework is seen as being able to identify the nurse's motivations and priorities by clearly defining the mode and parameters of nursing action.

Orem's self-care theory provides a conceptual framework within which to study phenomena uniquely related to practice situations in geriatric nursing care. An important feature of the theory is that it makes *explicit* the activity of the nurse in relation to the achievement of the care goal. It also defines the unique function of the professional nurse without usurping the central responsibility of the individual to work towards the achievement of an optimal level of self-care. Furthermore, in the geriatric ward situation, where the elderly person's independence and self-respect can be threatened so easily, the emphasis of the self-care theory on the achievement of an optimal level of self-care ensures that all types of elderly patients will be afforded the opportunity to aim towards the goal of optimal self-care. Optimal self-care is, therefore, a realistic aim for both remediable and long-stay patients, the difference being in the capacity of the individual's self-care potential.

A framework that describes appropriate modes of nursing action in relation to self-care potential may be more likely to achieve the right level of nursing assistance required to meet patients' needs. For those geriatric patients who are involved in rehabilitation, for example, the nurse's action would comprise guiding, supervising and teaching, while for certain long-stay patients, unable to perform particular self-care activities, nursing action would involve acting and doing for the patient. Figure 3 summarises the elements that make up the theorectical framework for geriatric nursing care.

## The self-care framework
The theoretical framework is conceptualised as consisting of three stages: the assessment, the nursing intervention or assistance stage and the outcome stage. At the assessment stage, data are collected relating to the universal, developmental and health deviational requirements of the individual and on how these are affecting his ability to provide self-care. Identification of any self-care demands experienced by the patient that are necessary to ensure an optimal health state is made at this point. These therapeutic self-care demands are then assessed in relation to the patient's own capacity to meet them; when the patient is unable to

GOAL CONTENTS

'Nursing seeks to achieve patient health or health related goals through self-care which is therapeutic; to overcome self-care deficits; and to foster and preserve self-care abilities of the patient.' (Nursing Development Conference Group, 1973, p.130)

PRESCRIPTION

Stage 1:  **Assessment**  1. *Self care agent:* assessment of factors that influence individuals' self-care ability
2. *Therapeutic self-care demands:*
   - universal
   - developmental
   - health deviational
3. *Self-care deficits:* areas of identified patient need for nursing assistance

Nursing diagnosis/plan of action

Stage 2:  **Assistance**  *Nursing*
*Assistance*                        *Nursing System*

1. Acting/doing         1. Wholly
   for                     compensatory
2. Guiding              2. Partially
3. Supporting             compensatory
4. Providing a         3. Supportive –
   therapeutic            educative
   environment
5. Teaching

Stage 3:  **Outcome**

Self-care              Therapeutic/optimal self-care

**Figure 3**  Theoretical framework for geriatric nursing care

meet his self-care needs a self-care deficit exists, and this is the responsibility of the nurse.

The nurse's mode of action is determined by specifying the most appropriate methods of nursing assistance. Depending on the extent and range of the individual's self-care deficits, coupled with the potential for recovery, the nurse may provide a wholly compensatory nursing care system in which she takes over most of the self-care activities of the patient. Alternatively, she may decide on the provision of a partially compensatory or supportive – educative nursing care system, in which the nurse's caring activities range from guidance, support and the provision of a therapeutic environment to teaching and supervising the patient in self-care activities.

Provision of the most approriate type of nursing action depends not only on the nurse's ability to assess patients' self-care needs but also on her level of knowledge, skill development and motivation to provide an individualised service according to the objective of the goal content. Nursing action may also be affected by the way in which nursing observations are operationalised into nursing activity. Within the self-care framework, the process of assessing, diagnosing, planning, implementing and evaluating nursing care is advocated (Joseph, 1980; Orem, 1980). Further influencing factors include the personal attibutes of both patient and nurse and also the environment within which the nursing action is performed.

An important feature of the system is that it focuses nursing attention on patients' self-care needs, thus legitimising the nurse's caring function rather than concentrating on the curing, medical model function. It also identifies the range of caring activities performed by the nurse, again not in relation to the medical needs of the patient, but in terms of assisting activities aimed specifically at the self-care abilities and deficits of the patient. The system recognises the fact that part of the nurse's role is that of an 'enabler' whose function is to help regain and maintain the patient's optimal independence, and this may involve the instruction and direction of significant others, e.g. the family or spouse, to provide care. The nurse would be provided with a clear indication of when the patient no longer requires her assistance, namely when he (or significant others) are capable of providing an optimal level of self-care that is therapeutic.

**Comparison of the self-care framework with Norton's geriatric nursing care model**

Whereas the model of geriatric nursing care identified in Norton's work (Norton et al, 1962; Norton, 1965) has served as a framework on which to analyse the development of nursing action, it was not considered to be the most appropriate or detailed model on which to base further analysis of the nurse's caring function. A brief comparison will be made of the similarities and differences between the original model and the proposed theoretical framework based on Orem's self-care concepts.

The main characteristics of a professional discipline have been discribed by Dickoff et al (1968). First, it is action-orientated, meaning that professionals shape reality according to an articulated purpose within the constraints of reality. Second, the professional has an important contribution to make in terms of interpreting and affecting the goal content. Figure 4 summarises the main similarities and differences between the self-care framework and Norton's model.

*Goal content*
According to the geriatric nursing care model, the outcome of the nurse's activity in the care of the elderly infirm is the discharge of remediable patients or the provision of basic nursing care to irremediable or long-stay patients. The goal content of the self-care theory framework, however, aims towards optimal self-care by the patient, so that he can achieve and maintain an optimal health state. The care goal is realised by the patient being encouraged to be as independent as possible in his self-care needs, whether he be in a long-stay ward, a rehabilitation ward in his own home.

*Prescription*
The geriatric nursing care model recognises the importance of accurately assessing each patient's nursing care needs, identifying nursing problems and providing means of solving such problems. Nursing action is viewed as being divided between meeting the needs of remediable and irremediable patients. For remediable patients the nurse's primary task is in the restoration of patients' self-care abilities, e.g. washing, feeding, dressing and elimination, with the gradual withdrawal of her assistance. In contrast, the

| Feature | Self-care framework (after Orem, 1971, 1980) | | Geriatric Nursing Care Model (after Norton et al, 1962) | |
|---|---|---|---|---|
| *Goal content* | Optimal self-care | | Recover of one's capacities; maintenance at optimal level of functioning | |
| *Prescription* | | | | |
| Assessment: | Self-care agent Therapeutic self-care demand   1. Universal self-care requisites   2. Developmental self-care     requisites   3. Health deviational     self-requisites | | Medical history Social history Nursing history | |
| Assistance | *Nursing* 1. Acting/doing   for 2. Guiding 3. Supporting 4. Providing a   therapeutic   environment 5. Teaching | *Nursing* 1. Wholly   compensatory   system 2. Partially   compensatory   system 3. Supportive   educative   system | *Remediable* Helping to rehabilitate the patient | *Irremediable* Acting/doing for; maintaining at optimal level |
| Outcome: | Goal:   Achievement of optimal level of   self-care for all patients | | Goal:   Gradual   withdrawal   support | Goal:   Maintenance   of patients at   optimal level   of functioning |

**Figure 4** Comparison of the theoretical framework for geriatric nursing care and the geriatric nursing care model

nurse's function in the care of irremediable patients is described as the 'provision of maximum comfort, happiness and peace of mind and maintaining an optimal level of functioning' (Norton, 1965).

The self-care theory framework identifies five main methods of nursing assistance, operationalised within three main nursing systems, the objective of each method being the provision of optimal self-care. The helping method chosen by the nurse is determined by the changing requirements of the patient. No distinction is made between remediable and irremediable patients as the patient's nursing needs would be classified according to the criteria laid down by the nursing systems identified.

| Variable | Self-care theory framework | | Geriatric nursing care model |
|---|---|---|---|
| The nurse | Knowledge<br>Skill<br>Motivation | | Knowledge<br>Skill<br>Attitude to elderly |
| The patient | *identification of:*<br>• universal<br>• developmental<br>  requirements<br>• health | | Defined according to<br>  medical diagnosis:<br>• remediable<br>• irremediable |
| The system of<br>nursing<br>care | Assessment<br>Diagnosis<br>Planning<br>Implementing<br>Evaluating | Process allows<br>  nurse to<br>  initiate,<br>  conduct and<br>  control<br>  assisting<br>  actions | Assessment<br>Planning<br>Monitor care through outcome<br>  nursing and individual care<br>  plans |
| Dynamics | Nursing action oriented – clear<br>  definition of nurse's goals,<br>  tasks and skills | | Nursing action based on<br>  medical definition of patients<br>  – remediable or irremediable<br>Nursing goals not clearly<br>  defined |

**Figure 5**   Variables by nursing care models as affecting nursing function

## Factors influencing the nurse's caring function

Both the geriatric care model and the self-care theory framework identify such factors as the environment, the organisational system and the lack of nursing knowledge and skills as potentially disruptive to the achievement of stated goals of care. Figure 5 summarises the main factors.

Although there are many similarities between the two frameworks (figures 4 and 5), the self-care framework is preferred for the following reasons. First, there is a more clearly articulated goal content, which is relevant to *all* geriatric patients, regardless of their medical prognosis. By having the goal content for all geriatric patient care as optimal self-care, the nurse is able to develop a range of assisting techniques. Second, the self-care framework provides clearer specification of nursing activity in both the assessment of patients' needs for nursing care and in the description of methods of nursing assistance. The self-care framework is also more able to consider the dynamics of the fluctuating needs of the patient, in that a patient defined according to a nursing system classification may be more likely to receive appropriate nursing assistance than is a patient who is defined according to medical model objectives. Finally, by virtue of a more clearly articulated goal content and by detailing the nurse's methods of assisting within particular nursing systems, the self-care model is thought to provide a more patient-centred service.

## The theoretical framework and the research design

Space has been devoted to the development of a theoretical framework for geriatric nursing care in oder both to identify the important elements of the nurse's task and to provide a framework for the design of the research study. Hirschfeld (1979, p.424) has commented on the importance of identifying a theoretical framework for geriatric nursing:

> 'An ... issue related to what kind of knowledge is looked for, lies in the choice of theoretical framework for research. The researcher must be aware that any theoretical framework will govern the findings to the extent that it guides and limits the observations made.'

The argument is that, instead of using a medical or social system framework, a nursing-based theoretical framework is needed to guide nursing research and practice. Research into the care of the hospitalised elderly (Towell, 1975; Baker, 1978; Evers, 1981a) has shown that differing methodological frameworks provide alternative perspectives on and interpretations of the problems that have been identified. An important consideration in evaluating the suitability of the theoretical framework is the extent to which it provides a nursing perspective that helps to define and explain the nurse's function. For example, although Evers (1981a) focused her analysis on the nursing care of hospitalised elderly patients, she chose to analyse the situation using a social systems approach, concentrating on the effect of the social relationship and interactions between the medical and nursing professions rather than directly attempting to analyse the nurse's caring function.

Baker (1978), who also used a social systems approach, decided to interpret the nurse's actions from a different standpoint, rejecting the predominant influence of social interaction on the nurse's function and concluding that nurses themselves, rather than the social system, were responsible for the hospitalised elderly and had to solve their problems. Evers (1982a,b) has commented on Baker's use of the social systems approach, noting that although Baker began by considering nursing within a social systems context, she ends up with an analysis bearing directly on the nurse's action and her perception of the situation. Evers feels that, within the theorectical framework described by Baker, the conclusions that Baker reaches do not fully concur with her social systems methodology.

By accepting the premise that the theoretical framework may guide and impose limits upon the observations made, it was decided to adopt a framework based on nursing principles. Such a framework would both define and direct the methodology, and would also serve as a basis upon which to analyse the observations and findings.

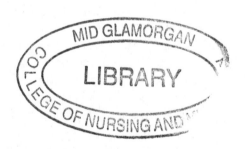

# 4 Study design

## INTRODUCTION

So far, the emphasis of the thesis has been on the need to identify a theoretical framework for geriatric nursing care with which to explain and direct nursing practice. Having identified the main theoretical concepts, the purpose of the study is to develop ways of applying such concepts to the practice setting in order to evaluate the nursing care being provided. It was decided to use a nursing framework rather than theoretical concepts from psychology or social sciences, despite the fact that few validated measures of nursing care exist that are based (explicity) on nursing theory. The researcher's first priority, therefore, was to develop appropriate measures that would reflect the underlying principles of the theory.

The orientation of the study design was based on two propositions; first that the majority of nurses have not fully recognised their caring function and, consequently, do not understand their role in the provision of nursing care for elderly patients; and, second, that a minority of nurses in geriatric care perceive their primary function to be the provision of patient-centred care, as opposed to routine-centred care. Leading on from this are two research questions:

1.  Can a composite measure based on theoretical concepts of nursing care be used to distinguish between different types of nursing action in geriatric wards, that is, nursing that is patient-centred (or therapeutic) and nursing action that is routine-centred (or less/non-therapeutic)?
2.  Can the same composite measure be used to identify methods of nursing activity that ensure patient-centred (or therapeutic) care?

The aim of the study design, therefore, was to provide a measure that would distinguish those nurses who were aware of their therapeutic function, as demonstrated by what they said and did, from those nurses who were less aware of their therapeutic function in the care of the elderly. The strength of the study design was felt to rest primarily on the way in which concepts of the theoretical framework were operationalised. In view of this, the steps involved in the construction, testing and development of the measure will be described in some detail. Chapters 5 and 6 deal with further aspects of the research design, which were dependent on the initial construction of the main measuring instrument.

## THE INSTRUMENT – A COMPOSITE INDICATOR

### Characteristics of indicators

When dealing with concepts such as quality of care, patient-centred care and optimal self-care, the researcher is immediately faced with the problem of quantifying such seemingly abstract and subjective observations in an objective and reliable way. Similar to the problems faced by social researchers in measuring quality of life or well-being are those confronting the nurse researcher who attempts to construct measures that reflect quality of nursing care. A series of research studies reported by McFarlane (1970) and Inman (1975) highlights some of the main methodological problems that arise from attempts to develop reliable criteria of care. On a wider perspective, Redfern (1981) documents the variety of approaches that have been used by researchers to develop ways of evaluating professional intervention and its effect on the quality of life and well-being of the elderly. Major problems uncovered by each of the studies in question include such factors as subjectivity, the questionable reliability of the tests and the multidimensionality of the concepts under scrutiny.

Despite the maze of methodological problems, the purpose of such measures is to act as indicators or pointers to phenomena that relate to the topic under investigation. For example, Redfern (1981, p.186) quotes Miller's (1978) study of the nursing care given in psychogeriatric wards to patients with dementia. Miller chose as an indicator of quality of nursing care a comparison of the amount of time patients were 'engaged' (i.e. the contact with people and/or manipulating moveable objects) with the amount of time they were 'disengaged' (i.e. when patients were isolated and given routine-type care). From her observations, Miller found that 41% of patients' time was spent 'engaged', whereas for 59% of the time patients were given more routine-type care. Miller concluded from this that more activities designed to increase the incidence of 'engaged' behaviour would improve patients' quality of life.

In a similar manner, Wells (1980, p.123) used the quality of nurse – patient verbal communication as an indicator of the quality of the nurse – patient relationship, demonstrating that neither were indicative of an acceptable standard of nursing care. Altschul (1972) and Stockwell (1972) have used the incidence of nurse – patient contact to demonstrate how nurses are influenced in their delivery of care by patient characteristics, whereas other researchers have used physical, psychological and social indicators to demonstrate the link between nursing action and quality of care. Examples of the latter include: the use of physiological reactions to anxiety as an indicator of the patients' postoperative experiences (Boore, 1978); psychological reaction to postoperative pain, and how this is affected by nursing support and the provision of information at the preoperative stage (Hayward, 1975); and studies of the effectiveness of domicilary nursing in relation to social and economic functioning (Skeet, 1970; Parnell and Naylor, 1973).

An important feature of such measurement techniques is the need to link them with wider theory. From the social theory perspective, Land (1971) has argued that social indicators should be seen as components within a sociological model of a social system, thereby making indicators more than just some sort of statistical series. Hockey (1977) gives a reminder that indicators are tools and, as such, they are a means to an end and not ends in themselves. Thus, the purpose and objective of the indicator must be recognised before its usefulness can be appraised (Hockey, 1977, p.239). In addition, given the variety of factors that could be used as indicators, Hockey (1977, p.243) feels that of fundamental importance to the choice of suitable indicators is the explicit declaration of one's theoretical frame of reference.

Indicators have been defined by Carlisle (1972, p.25) as 'the operational definitions or part of the operational definition of any of the concepts central to the generation of an information system, descriptive of the (social) system'. She goes on to identify central concepts of the social system that must be operationalised through the indicator if it is to be a fair reflection of the components of the theoretical framework. These include system components, system goals, problem areas and system objectives. Carlisle also points out that the way in which these concepts are operationalised will affect the accuracy of the methodology. They must be operationalised in such way that they can be related back to the unmeasurable concepts of which they are representations as well as being 'concrete' enough to be easily quantifiable.

Brand (1975), however, suggests that it is rather illogical to believe that unquantifiable information is of less importance than that which can be quantified. He feels that the researcher must be able to deal with indirectly measurable, subjective variables in the process of quantitative data analysis, arguing that although this introduces additional unknowns into the system, those unknowns have, in any event, always been implicitly present. The implications of this are such that, in the initial development of an indicator of nursing care, a whole range of factors must be considered that reflect the extent of the concepts under scrutiny.

In addition to the need for close links between indicators and the theoretical concepts of which they are representations – both quantitative and on a more intuitive or subjective level – Carley (1981) underlines the importance of ensuring that the research design consists of methodologically appropriate techniques that do not ignore certain scientific criteria. He suggests that attention be given in the overall design to such problems as quantification, the effect of value judgments internal to the analysis, prediction and causality. A further problem in the research design is related to indicator selection. Often, there is such a wide range of output (observable data) that may be associated with a particular dependent variable that the observed strength of the relationship may consequently be diluted. Increasing the number of indicators in order to have one check another is not a good guarantee that each and every one is not a poor indicator (Bunge, 1975, p.69). When the phenomena under scrutiny are complex and multidimensional (as in the case in quality of nursing care studies), a composite range of indicators is often necessary to relfect accurately such measures as quality of care. There is often a poor correlation between objective nursing indicators and the individuals's perceived quality of care, and this, together with the need for comprehensive cover of the contributing factors, sometimes leads to the presentation of too many measures. One way round this is to define a manageable number of variables, which are directly linked to the central concepts of the underlying theory. A group of such indicators can be used as a composite index. This method of quantification using a group of simple indicators is thought to be more useful than using a multitude of individual indicators (Carley, 1981, p.79). The main requirement of a composite index is that unlike measures can be transformed into a common scale so that they can be added together (this process may be followed by value weighting).

Given the nature of the research problem, which was to test whether a measure based on nursing concepts of care could be used to explain nursing action, it was decided to adopt a methodology based on the construction and use of a composite nursing indicator called the Therapeutic Nursing Function or TNF indicator. The indicator is based on the theoretical framework for geriatric nursing care described earlier, and centres attention on the specific contribution of the nurse in the particular situation.

**The TNF indicator – theoretical components**

Central to the nursing theory advocated in this thesis are the two principles of nursing as a caring activity and geriatric care as the positive approach to the health and welfare of the elderly infirm. These principles were given more substance and direction by the adoption of Orem's (1980) self-care framework, which provided a system of evaluating nursing care based on the goal of optimal self-care or independence. The goal was translated into reality by means of an elaborate prescription of nursing activities based on the provision of patient-centred care (see figure 3 above). Both the nurse and the patient were seen as important contributors to the overall success of the interaction, as were a variety of organizational and environmental factors that might affect the outcome.

Using theoretical features identified by Dickoff et al (1968), the main concepts of the theoretical framework pertaining to the operationalisation process were identified as the goal content, the prescription and the survey list. The goal content (which is equivalent to Carlisle's system and policy goals) must be identifiable within the practice setting, either in terms of action or of what the nurse describes as her goals of care. The prescription, which equates with Carlisle's system components and objectives, provides information as to the organisation and management of care within the practice setting. The method of organisation and management advocated by the theoretical model is based on individualised patient care, in which nurses are responsible for assessing, planning, implementing and evaluating their care within the goal of optimising self-care. Features of the survey list (problem areas) include those extraneous variables within the system that must be considered in the process of working toward optimal self-care. In addition to the organisation system, account must be taken of such features as the environment, the patients' characteristics and the nurse's personal characteristics.

Another feature of the theoretical framework, which was identified as being important in the development of the research design, was the deliberate orientation of the indicator to describe and evaluate nursing action rather than patient action or experiences. The decision to concentrate on the nurse, and particularly the activities and opinions of the ward sister, was made for a number of reasons. Most importantly, the decision to concentrate on nurses rather than patients was based on the proposition that nurses have not internalised their caring function and, consequently, do not fully understand their role in the provision of care to elderly patients. Furthermore, one of the main features of the theoretical framework based on Orem's self-care concept was the detailed description of the nurse's activities in relation to the self-care needs of her patients. Here, the nurse determines the nature of her nursing intervention in relation to the patient's need for assistance. Accordingly, the nurse is not only deciding what method of assistance to use but also assessing the patient's actual and potential need for care.

The ability of the nurse to decide how to use her skills, abilities and knowledge in each nursing situation was considered to be an important component in the whole theoretical framework and, as such, was termed the nurse's therapeutic function.

## The nurse's therapeutic function

The term 'therapeutic' has been linked with the activities of health-care professionals for many years, notably in the areas of therapeutics and rehabilitation and in several branches of psychiatry. From the nursing perspective, Travelbee's (1977) description of the nurse as a therapeutic agent is perhaps the most enlightening. She begins by stating that as well as acquiring appropriate knowledge and skills, the nurse needs to be able to use *herself therapeutically* in order to provide nursing care. Travelbee (1977, p.25) goes on to explain what the term means:

> 'When a nurse uses self therapeutically she consciously makes use of her personality and knowledge in order to effect a change in the ill person. This change is considered therapeutic when it alleviates the individual's distress.'

Travelbee (p.45) also states that the quality of nursing care given to any person is determined by the nurse's perception of the ill person and the nurse's beliefs about human beings. Thus, from a nursing point of view, therapeutic action comprises both emotional and personal interaction as well as the use of knowledge and skills. Peplau (1952) and Lewis (1966) believe that the kind of person the nurse becomes influences the quality and quantity of learning that takes place in the patients she is nursing, whereas Uys (1980, p.175) holds that when the nurse is aware of her therapeutic effect on the patient, she can scientifically and purposefully employ her entire person or a combination of her personality elements to act as a tool for promoting health and limiting disease.

Hardy (1982) contends that failure to consider this facet of the nurse's contribution to patient care has led to restrictive views of nursing models of practice. She identifies two areas that she feels have been overlooked by the majority of nurse theorists such as Abdellah et al (1960), Riehl and Roy (1980) and King (1981), to the detriment of nurse knowledge and nurse action. These include acknowledgement of the nurse's ability to use herself therapeutically in the nursing situation, an activity which involves the nurse in a more personal exchange with the patient, and the need to identify the content and scope of nursing skills and nursing knowledge.

The important concepts identified as characteristics of the nurse's therapeutic function also reflect components of Griffin's (1980, 1983) concept of care. Intermingled with the structural components of organising a system of nursing care, managing that system and ensuring the proper channels of communication, is the need to respond, to feel, to comfort and to care. For a nursing activity to be seen as therapeutic – or to have elements of therapeutic activity in it – the nurse must be in a system that allows her to organise the structural components in such a way that she is free to interact in a more personal – and therapeutic – way with her patients. The main structural components that are thought to influence the therapeutic potential of the nurse are documented in the theoretical framework (see figure 3 above) and must be considered in any analysis of the nurse's therapeutic awareness. These include such features as the goal content, the organisation of work on the ward and any extraneous variables that may impede the nurse. From the more interpersonal perspective, the nurse's therapeutic function is indicated by her ability to use her personality, knowledge and skills in such a way that she can effect a positive change in the condition of the patient. Such interpersonal components of the nurse's therapeutic function may be measured using such indicators as her opinions or level of skill utilisation, her knowledge base, her understanding of the needs of the patients or her attitudes, and also by observing her interactions with the patient.

Thus, in the process of identifying and refining the main components of the nursing indicator that will be used as a measure of quality of care, it was thought impossible to consider patient care without recognising the impact of the nurse's therapeutic contribution to the system. Such a therapeutic contribution would involve the provision of nursing assistance in a way that would ensure the dignity and optimal independence of the patient. Achieving this goal would also be dependent on an organisational system that would allow the nurse to carry out individualised patient care within an environment that would optimize self-care and patient independence. In such settings, the nurse could use a range of nursing assistance techniques, from doing everything for the patient to supervising, encouraging or teaching the patient. It was within such a conceptual arrangement that the composite indicator – the TNF indicator – was constructed.

## CONSTRUCTION OF THE TNF INDICATOR

The construction of the indicator was complex, in that nursing activity was seen to involve a range of factors comprising such concepts as attitudes, values, motivation, action, knowledge and skill. These were evaluated in terms of the nurse's perception of geriatric care (goal content), her mode of organising and managing the work (prescription) and her documented level of skill utility and knowledge of care of the elderly (aspects of the survey list). It was decided to concentrate on the construction of a composite index, which incorporated the above factors. These were reflections of the theoretical framework and, if performed by the nurse in a manner that guaranteed optimal self-care, were regarded as therapeutic.

## Practical aspects involved in the construction of the TNF indicator

The final configuration of the TNF indicator depended on the three main factors: that theoretical concepts were observable and measurable; that the indicator would be administered to a representative sample population of nurses in Northern Ireland; and that the indicator was both a reliable and valid measure of the concepts under investigation. Figure 6 summarises the central concepts of the nursing theory, which were operationalised by means of the TNF indicator. It also describes the type of instrumentation used, a more detailed account of which is given in appendices I and II. In the discussion that follows, the main components of figure 6 are described in detail, thereby explaining the operationalisation of the theoretical concepts and attempting to justify the indicator in terms of its reliability and validity. As far as the researcher's choice of sample population is concerned, suffice it to say at this moment, that, after considering possibility of using all grades of nurse to measure the level of TNF awareness, a decision was made to concentrate on ward sisters, for the following reasons. First, it was felt that ward sisters were best equipped to answer questions on how information is gathered, processed and implemented on their ward, and, second, the organisational priorities of the ward sister have been shown to be influential factors in the way information is collected on wards. As such, the sister's attitudes and actions have an influence on the way in which nursing staff perform their jobs (Pembrey, 1980, p.26). Other studies have demonstrated that the ward sister also commands a significantly influential position, not only in organising and managing ward work but also in teaching and encouraging ward staff (Baker, 1978; Fretwell, 1978; Orton, 1979)

| Main concepts | Operational definition | Instrument |
|---|---|---|
| 1. Goal content of care/perception of work | 1. Nurse's definition for geriatric nursing | Open-ended question |
| | 2. Proportion of time spent on basic nursing care activities | Ranking of 8 items in order of priority |
| | 3. Allocation of time according to nursing priorities | Ranking of 8 items in order of priority |
| 2. Prescription/ organisational and planning of nursing care | 1. Method of organising nursing care on ward | Set of 11 structured questions asking ward sisters to state methods/system most like their own |
| | 2. Evidence of an 'active management cycle' | Set of 5 questions based on Pembrey's (1980) identification of 'manager' and 'non-manager' sisters |
| 3. Survey list/variables that may affect the nurse's activity | 1. Knowledge | Open-ended/structured questions about the level of nurse training and opinions as to its effectiveness |
| | 2. Skill utilisation/work choice/level of satisfaction | Structured questions relating to nurses' awareness of their skills and opinions as to their level of skill utilisation |
| | 3. Perception of rehabilitation role | Open-ended question of nurse's description and understanding of her role in the rehabilitation of patients |

**Figure 6** Operationalisation of central concepts of nursing theory in construction of the indicator

and in acting as a positive role model for younger staff nurses and students (Fretwell, 1978).

*Goal content*
The nurse's definition of geriatric nursing was thought to be a useful indicator of nursing action in that the way the nurse perceives her work reflects her methods of action (Towell, 1975;

Evers, 1981a). This has also been clearly demonstrated by Baker (1978), who identified two main types of nurse action that were related to the nurse's perception of geriatric patients. The predominant type was routine-style geriatric nursing care, which was geared principally to the undifferentiated distribution of impersonal, basic care to patients who, according to Baker's analysis, were seen as less than whole and usual persons and whose needs were regarded as secondary to those of nurse managers and staff. Nurses viewed such patients as requiring nothing more than the provision of a minimal level of physical care, and they described their nursing in terms of overwhelming time-consuming activities of daily life (Baker, 1978, p.102). In contrast, a minority of nurses, the second category, were found to emphasise the need to treat patients as responsible adults, involving them as far as possible in decisions about their lives. This approach underlined the nurse's belief that the elderly person was a whole and usual person, as distinct from a tainted and discounted one. Baker found that this attitude was observable in the nurse's perception of her caring role, where she described her function in relation to patient rehabilitation and where all nursing activities concerned with direct patient care were based on an assessment of the patient's individual needs.

By asking the nurse to define geriatric nursing, it was hoped to obtain some indication of what she thought of her role, whether it centred on the provision of individualised care to patients who were viewed as 'whole and usual' people or whether her role was more involved with the provision of routine, basic nursing care. Appendix I, part 1, question 1, gives the format of the question, while appendix II shows the scale used to measure the level of therapeutic awareness of the ward sister in this area. This scale was constructed using Baker's (1978) observations as a basis.

An example of a nursing definition that was given a top rating of 5 on the scale is:

'Q. What does geriatric nursing involve?

A. It involves having a genuine caring attitude, seeing the patients as individuals, being progressive enough to make alterations on the ward to provide a therapeutic environment and homely atmosphere for the individual. It involves ensuring patient safety without over-protection, a high degree of nurse-relative involvement and being able to understand those who have communication difficulties.' (Ward Sister, geriatric ward)

In contrast, a reply that was given a bottom rating of 1 on the scale described geriatric nursing in the following way:

> 'Caring for the physical needs of patients, keeping them clean and comfortable.' (Ward Sister, geriatric ward)

Linked with the ward sister's definition of geriatric care were two structured questions (see figure 6 and appendices I and II) asking the ward sister to indicate her priorities of care in terms of how she spent her time on the ward and how she rated certain activities in order of importance. The decision to include such a question came from observations made by Rhys Hearn (1979a,b) and Norwich (1980), who noted that despite being provided with optimal numbers of staff to carry out patient-centred activities, nurses chose to spend additional time they had in the performance of routine, physical care activities. By asking the ward sister to state first, the time she spent on certain activities (broadly divided into basic nursing care and more patient-focused care, e.g. communication, exercising, toilet-training rather than dealing with incontinence), areas of nursing activity that the ward sister felt were most important could be ascertained. A complementary question asked the ward sister to rank certain activities in order of importance, which broadly reflected a basic nursing care approach, a medical model approach and a total patient or individualised patient care approach to nursing. (See appendices I and II, questions 2 and 3.)

*Prescription*
Two main areas were covered in the prescription stage of the TNF indicator (see figure 6). These were a consideration of the extent to which the ward sister had a system of individualised patient care operating on her ward, and an assessment of whether she actively managed the ward situation. These features have been shown to be integral components of a patient-centred approach to nursing care (Baker, 1978; Grant, 1979; Pembrey, 1980). Grant (1979, p.30), for example, states that individualised care can be defined as an 'ideology of management of care of a person on the basis of his unique needs, the objective being maximum independence from the necessity of such care'. She sees the nurse's responsibility to individualised patient care as including an attempt to understand the patient's perception of his need for nursing assistance and to function on the basis of that perception. Grant also identifies the

nurse's role as embracing counselling, teaching, supervising and assisting activities, all based within the managerial framework of individualised patient care.

Grant (1979, pp.30–44) identified the nursing care plan or the individual care plan assessment as the vehicle through which patient-centred care could be operationalised in the ward setting. From her observations, several aims of the individual care plan assessment were identified that would help to evaluate the degree to which ward sisters in geriatric wards attempted to provide patient-centred care. These included a description of the extent of the patient's history: whether or not it included social, psychological and emotional aspects as well as medical information and activities of living capacity. The clarity with which the whole patient data gathering system was explained by the ward sister was also thought to indicate how it was used in the ward. The ward sister's description of how nursing staff were provided with information about patients was also thought to reflect the type of patient management system in operation. This included such areas as finding out how accessible the information collected from patients was to nursing staff, whether or not it was used, how the information was used to construct nursing care plans, whether or not time limits were set in the monitoring of patient problems and how goals were reassessed (appendix I, section 2).

Grading of the responses given by ward sisters to this series of questions was based on information about individualised care planning taken from Hunt and Marks-Maran (1980), Little and Carnevali (1969), Mayers (1978), Grant (1979) and Yura and Walsh (1973). Figure 7 shows how the series of questions comprising the instrument was based on the nursing process framework. This list of questions (appendix I, section 2) attempted to cover each important area detailed in figure 7, whereas the scaling techniques outlined in appendix 2, section 2 provided a means by which the responses could be graded according to patient-centred (or therapeutic) or routine-type care orientation.

The second component in the prescription phase of the TNF indicator assessed the degree to which the ward sister actually managed the nursing care on her ward. Identification of an active management cycle in nursing was carried out by Pembrey (1980), who believed that the ward sister was the crucial agent in determining the form of work organization in the ward, which either enabled nurses to nurse patients or prevented them from

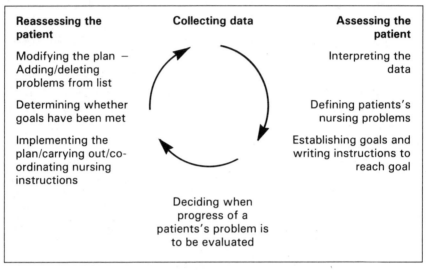

| Reassessing the patient | Collecting data | Assessing the patient |
|---|---|---|
| Modifying the plan – Adding/deleting problems from list | | Interpreting the data |
| Determining whether goals have been met | | Defining patients's nursing problems |
| Implementing the plan/carrying out/co-ordinating nursing instructions | | Establishing goals and writing instructions to reach goal |
| | Deciding when progress of a patients's problem is to be evaluated | |

**Figure 7**  Components of patient-centred (therapeutic) care (from: Hunt and Marks-Maran, 1980)

doing so. She identified several types of critical behaviour required of the ward sister in relation to the active daily management of nursing. These included the delegation of authority to individual nurses to exercise discretion (within prescribed limits) and the subsequent exacting of accountability from nurses to ensure that nursing had been achieved. Pembrey (1980, p.58) was then able to construct a 'degree of management continuum', which placed individualised patient care and individual nurse responsibility at one end (the 'management' end), whereas the 'non-management' extreme were non-individualised patient care and task allocation.

The ward sister's position on the management continuum was based on her activities in relation to the nursing management cycle, which comprised information on how the ward sister identified the ward workload, how she prescribed work (both written and verbally), how she delegated authority in the allocation of nursing staff on the ward and the way in which she exacted accountability for the work done by the nurses. (See appendix I, section 2b for the question format, and appendix II, section 2b for the scaling method.) An active management cycle in which the ward sister completely performed each of the aspects classified on the continuum was shown to relate directly to an awareness on the ward sister's part of her therapeutic function. Both the active management cycle indicator and the TNF scale are based on Pembrey's (1980) analysis of ward sisters. Pembrey demonstrated how an active management approach was a pre-requisite for the provision of patient-centred or therapeutic nursing care.

*Survey list – knowledge and skills*
Included in the TNF indicator was a series of questions relating to the survey list. An attempt was made to find out what ward sisters thought both of their training for geriatric care and of their skill repertoire. In a recent geriatric textbook, Irvine et al (1978) have documented important components of the nurse's knowledge and skills. As far as the nurse's knowledge base is concerned, they believe she ought to understand something of the process of ageing, the presentation of disease in old age and the problems of multiple disability. She must also understand something of the workings of community service for the elderly and the organisation of the geriatric unit, and appreciate the value of specialised equipment and the importance of good ward design for the elderly. In relation to skill acquisition, Irvine et al (1978, p.43) stress the importance of the 'traditional' skills, together with the ability to help the patient help himself, stating that 'in geriatric training the nurse will learn how to withdraw her assistance to enable the patient to do more on his own.'

Wells' (1980) study of geriatric nurses found, however, that in practice their knowledge of the problems confronting the elderly was very poor. Wells highlighted the need for a comprehensive in-service education programme for both trained and untrained staff. Wells also noted (1980, p.46) with alarm, the fact that some of the suggestions put forward by staff as problem-solving techniques were 'global, vague and reflected a possible lack of knowledge of anatomy and physiology'.

The proposition in the present study was that those ward sisters who were more aware of their therapeutic function would identify their need (and the profession's) for more detailed and com-prehensive training in geriatric nursing care (appendix I, section 3). Ward sisters' responses were scaled according to their perception of the need for more training, the top grading being given where the respondent listed at least three areas in which more knowledge was required (appendix II, section 3).

The TNF indicator assessed the ward sister's opinion of the way in which her nursing skills were being used, particularly the ward sister's description of her rehabilitation function (appendices I and II, section 3). This series of questions was based on an idea from Hockey (1976), who found that nurses' level of skill utilisation was related to their level of job satisfaction. Given the fact that a common description of geriatric nursing comprises just 'good basic nursing care', the researcher was interested to see whether ward sisters felt they had more than just the 'traditional' nursing care skills. Ward sisters who felt that very good use was being made of each of the named skills were rated as having a high TNF score, whereas those ward sisters who felt little use was being made of their skills were given a lower score. Two additional questions at this point asked for details as to the ward sister's motivation for working on a geriatric ward and the aspects of the job that ward sisters found most enjoyable. These questions were included to help determine whether ward sisters were content with their work (appendix II, section 3).

The final set of questions dealt with the ward sister's understanding of the concept of rehabilitation. The researcher was keen to find out what ward sisters understood by this term, i.e. whether it was defined by the ward sister from a medical model perspective or from a nursing point of view. The nursing conception of rehabilitation was thought to have been best described by Norton (1965), who defined the nurse's action in terms of 'reabling' remedial patients by supporting, assisting and encouraging them to regain their independence, and by maintaining at their optimal level of self-care those patients whom Norton termed irremedial or continuing care patients. Thus, the therapeutic content of the ward sister's rehabilitation role was based on the extent to which she saw her role as one of facilitator and being able to maintain her patient at the optimal level of self-care. Examples of the components of responses that were classed as therapeutic are given in appendix II, section 3.

## The TNF indicator – comments and considerations

Thus far, a primary aim of the research project had been met, in that a nursing measurement instrument had been constructed from theoretical perspectives based on the concept of care. Whereas the theoretical approach could guarantee a degree of content validity, the indicator had yet to be proved to be an accurate measure of nursing activity in the ward setting. The next stage of the study design, therefore, involved the testing of the TNF indicator to see whether it could distinguish between nursing action that was patient-centred (or therapeutic) and nursing action that was routine-centred. If the indicator proved capable of distinguishing between these two types of nursing action, the study could progress to assessment of the reliability and validity of the instrument.

In endeavouring to develop a suitable methodology, a number of factors had to be considered. First, because the indicator was a new construct, developed from a nursing theoretical framework, there were few guidelines as to the best or most appropriate way of testing the instrument in the practice setting. Second, the TNF indicator encompassed a wide range of conceptual areas, from perceptions of nursing and ideas about rehabilitation to methods of ward organisation and staff deployment. Although each area could have merited a study in its own right, an assumption had to be made that, in terms of the TNF indicator, each area was of equal importance to the final manifestation of nursing action. Because such an assumption was made, it was considered inappropriate to employ a methodological approach using measures whose reliability and validity would have to be already accepted. As such claims could not be made about the TNF indicator, the study design rested on the presentation of a descriptive and observational account of the application of the measurement instrument in the research area.

Another assumption involved the acceptance of the theoretical framework. This would be used as a yardstick in the analysis of ward observations, and projections made from it would be used as the criteria upon which to base the interpretation of results. In the development of the study design, it was assumed that one could legitimately measure deviations from the theoretical concepts operationalised in the TNF indicator, by comparing the hypothetical action of the patient-centred or therapeutic ward sister with the actual response. Quantification of these responses involved placing a numerical value on the TNF indicator responses, which graded them in relation to their deviation from the guidelines of the theoretical model.

A fourth consideration concerned the way in which the numerical data were to be handled. As a composite measure, the indicator had to evaluate each area of observation on a common scale. An ordinal-type scale was developed, which grouped responses into predetermined categories relating to the level of TNF awareness. Because the numerical data could not be interpreted in strict quantitative terms, the final scores were taken as indications of the general orientation of the respondents to either end of the TNF scale. Statistical measures such as medians and interquartile ranges, rather than any of the range of inferential statistics, which would assume certain quantitative features of the numerical data, were used to identify groups of respondents.

Given such constraints, a more descriptive and observational approach to the study design was adopted. This was preferred not only because of the constraints imposed by the TNF indicator but also because very little descriptive information was found to exist on the state of geriatric nursing in Northern Ireland. The lack of general descriptive information, together with the need to test the indicator in as representative a way as possible, pointed to the choice of a social survey approach to testing the indicator. This would involve consideration of the total population of geriatric ward facilities, from which a representation sample could be randomly selected. It also permitted the inclusion of a range of extraneous variables, such as the ward environment, patient characteristics and general descriptive information about nursing staff, that were considered to be important in the overall analysis.

Whereas the social survey approach could provide general descriptive data on ward sisters' level of TNF awareness and on a range of extraneous variables, it was restricted in its ability to evaluate certain aspects of the TNF indicator, particularly how the opinions and actions of the ward sister would actually affect the patients' experience of care on the ward. Thus, as an extension to testing the TNF indicator by standard social survey techniques, a further study was planned to describe aspects of the TNF indicator in a more detailed and personal way. This consisted of a comparative case-study approach, in which the nursing activity in a ward whose ward sister had been identified as having a high TNF score (and was, therefore, assumed to be therapeutic or patient-centred in her approach to care) was compared to the nursing activity observed on a ward whose ward sister obtained a low TNF score (which was assumed to be an indicator of routine-centred or non-therapeutic care). The case-study approach would involve observation of nursing action in each ward over a prescribed time period. If there was a significant difference between the quantity and quality of care given in the two wards, this would help to validate the TNF indicator as a predictive measure of the quality of nursing care. A brief outline of the two phases of the study design will be given, detailed explanation of the methodology and results being found in the following chapters.

## TESTING THE INDICATOR

### The social survey approach

The main considerations in this phase of the study design were the choice of a representative sample of geriatric wards, the development of a method by which to administer the TNF indicator and the development of a range of measurement instruments that would gather information on areas such as ward layout and facilities, patient characteristics, paramedical coverage and demographic information on nursing staff working on the wards.

### *Sampling*
The basic sampling unit could have been either the ward sister or the geriatric ward, but by using the geriatric ward as the sampling unit, it was considered that information about the total population could be obtained more easily. In addition, the primary sampling unit could be used as a cluster sample to select ward sisters, patients and nurses. Other factors taken into account included the way in which the total population was to be defined, the methods of collecting the most up-to-date sampling list, the choice of sampling technique and the method of obtaining permission to use the randomly selected sample units.

### *Measurement instruments*
Having identified a number of important areas of data collection supplementary to the TNF indicator, a major task of this phase was to develop appropriate measurement instruments, which could be distributed easily to a sample of geriatric wards across the Province, and three main measurement instruments were developed. These were a Ward Survey Form, a Patient Status Form and a Staff Questionnaire. The Ward Survey Form included

two main sections. The first section was an interview schedule designed to obtain information from the ward sister about aspects of the ward environment. The second section consisted of a Ward Survey List, used to detail information on the physical layout of the ward and on the range of furniture and equipment in use. A Ward Profile Scale was used to evaluate the observations made from the Ward Survey List.

The Patient Status Form was devised as a measure of patients' functional mobility and self-care abilities. Based on an assessment form documented by Barrowclough and Pinel (1979), staff were asked to grade the levels of mobility and functional ability of their patients. The final measurement instrument was the Staff Questionnaire, in which were contained the TNF indicator questions. The aims of the questionnaire were two-fold. First, and more importantly, the questionnaire was designed to obtain information from all ward sisters on their level of therapeutic activity. The questionnaire was divided into three main sections dealing with demographic information, levels of job satisfaction and nurses' comments and perceptions of their work. The indicator questions were distributed throughout these three sections, each section containing those questions pertaining to it. This distribution made it more difficult for ward sisters to identify the key questions. The questionnaire also contained questions that could be answered by all nursing staff, and by their so doing, it was hoped to build up a more comprehensive picture of nursing on geriatric wards.

Questionnaires were designed to be self-administered, thus ensuring that as wide a sample of staff as possible could be reached within the time available.

The main objectives of the survey stage were to provide information about the TNF indicator and to provide descriptive data on the range of extraneous variables that may have an influence on the ward sister's TNF indicator score. The effect of such variables could only be speculative, given the methods of data analysis. However, such observations were considered to be important to the overall discussion of the utility of the TNF indicator as a measure of quality of nursing care.

# DEVELOPING THE INDICATOR

In the final stage, the study design moved from a wide-scale social survey approach to a more detailed, comparative case-study approach, in which the activities of nurses in two ward situations were observed and analysed. A brief explanation of why this approach was adopted will be followed by an outline of the measurement instruments developed.

## The case-study approach – rationale

It was intended that the TNF indicator, in conjunction with the descriptive and observational data collected during the survey stage, would be able to distinguish ward sisters whose stated approach to their work was therapeutic or patient-centred (at the top end of the TNF indicator scale) and ward sisters whose approach was less therapeutic or routine-centred (at the lower end of the scale). As an additional step towards testing the 'correctness' of such classifications, it was decided to undertake an in-depth study of the nursing care given to a group of patients in one ward at the top end of the scale, and to compare these results with the nursing care given to a group of patients in a ward whose ward sister's TNF score was at the lower end of the scale.

Such an investigation was considered possible using a comparative case-study approach in which representativeness (a feature of the social survey approach) would be substituted for depth of analysis. By using the case-study approach, it would also be possible to develop particular areas of interest identified by the survey approach, which, because of the lack of detailed information, it had not been possible to discuss analytically. This more detailed, in-depth analysis of the nursing care of geriatric patients was seen as an important and necessary dimension to the study design, particularly given the fact that data analysis was based on description and observation of situations, using the theoretical framework as a yardstick.

## Outline of measurement instruments

The choice of wards would depend on the results obtained from the TNF indicator. The researcher also considered whether certain extraneous variables, such as ward facilities and paramedical cover, ought not to be controlled in the case-study approach. Again, a decision could be made only after the results of the TNF indictor had been analysed. What could be considered at this stage was the type of instrumentation to be used in collecting data. However, before instruments could be devised, the main areas of investigation in the ward situation had to be identified. This was achieved by using the same theoretical framework as had been used in the construction of the TNF indicator. The common objective of each instrument was to identify the extent to which the main elements of the TNF indicator, that is, the goal content, prescription and survey list, were being operationalised in the ward situation (see figure 8).

Providing information on the TNF indicator in an observational and quantifiable way involved first the collection of information about the nursing assessment and nursing care plan of patients on the wards being observed. Analysis of the nursing assessment would focus on information relating to: the patients' self-care agency, i.e. the baseline level of self-care and the level of functioning as it related to universal, developmental and health deviational self-care requirements; the self-care deficits, i.e. areas in which the patient was unable to meet his self-care needs; and the therapeutic self-care demand, i.e. the type of nursing assistance required to meet the patient's self-care needs. Patients' individual nursing care plans would also be examined to see whether distinct nursing goals had been identified and, if so, whether or not clear instructions were given to meet such goals.

The evaluation of written nursing information, using the parameters of the theoretical framework, was used as a baseline with which to judge nurse – patient interaction on the ward. Outcomes of observed nurse – patient interaction were compared to the prescribed or projected outcomes identified in the written information. In order to achieve this, some method of observing and recording a range of nurse – patient interactions had to be developed.

The final area that required documentation was linked to the opinions of the nurses being observed. It was felt that having an instrument which ensured that staff on the ward had the opportunity to comment on their impressions of how work was organised and on what they thought about how the nursing care they provided would be a useful means of evaluating the impact

| TNF indicator main concepts | Operational definition | Aspects of nursing function | Measurement instruments |
|---|---|---|---|
| *Goal content* | Perception of geriatric nursing | Achieving optimal patient independence/self-care through deliberate and purposeful nursing action | Patient goal identification (written) Non-participation observation of nursing care of elderly patients |
| *Prescription* | Patient information system | Accurate nursing assessment Nursing care planning Identification of patient problems Setting of nursing goals Evaluation of nursing outcomes | Evaluation of written nursing information on ward |
| | Active management cycle | Communication nursing information Documentation of patient information Delegation of work Work accountability | Observation of nurses Semi-structured interviews with staff |
| *Survey list* | Knowledge Skills | *Nursing action* 1. Acting/doing for 2. Guiding/supporting 3. Supervising 4. Providing therapeutic environment 5. Teaching  *Nursing systems* 1. Wholly compensatory 2. Partly compensatory 3. Supportive – educative | Intermittent non-participant observation of 8 patients in geriatric wards |

**Figure 8**  Outline of theoretical development of the TNF indicator

of the prescription system in operation on the ward.

Three main measurement instruments were, therefore, developed to cover these areas: an instrument based on the theoretical framework that evaluated written nursing information; a semi-structured interview schedule for ward staff; and the use of intermittent, non-participant observation techniques to obtain information on nurse–patient interaction.

## Evaluation of written information

Information about patients' nursing care requirements came from a variety of sources: from medical notes, the nursing Kardex and care plan and paramedical notes. Using the parameters identified by the theoretical framework, the researcher could use patients' information to determine their self-care potential and, hence, goal content. This also provided a means of categorising patients into one of the three main nursing systems: wholly compensatory, partly compensatory and supportive–educative. These were linked with the most appropriate type of nursing assistance required by the patient in order to achieve the stated care goals and meet the therapeutic self-care demand.

The collection of written information in the case study served three main purposes. First, it provided the researcher with background information of patients' level of self-care and their need for nursing assistance. Second, it allowed patients to be divided into three groups, depending on their need for nursing assistance. Third, the collection and assessment of such information enabled the researcher to draw conclusions about the goal content and the methods of work prescription on the ward.

## Staff interviews

In the testing of the TNF indicator, ward sisters had been asked to describe how they delegated and controlled work on the ward. An assumption, substantiated by the research of Pembrey (1980), had been made linking the extent to which the ward sister actively managed her ward with the level of patient-centred (or therapeutic) care given. A similar assumption was made in the case study: namely that nurses in a ward where the sister actively managed patient care would be more likely to provide patient-centred care than would nurses in a ward where the sister did not actively manage the work. The main objective of the staff interviews was to ascertain what each of the nurses in the ward thought about how their work was organised, and whether or not they felt it allowed them to provide patient-centred care. A semi-structured staff interview schedule was used by the researcher as a means of directing and controlling the interview (see appendix IXe in Kitson, 1984).

*Intermittent non-participant observation*

The final measurement instrument involved the development of a method of evaluating the quantity and quality of nurse – patient interaction. The main aim of the non-participant observation was to document the frequency and quality of the interactions between the nurse and the patient. Eight patients were chosen on each ward and nursing interaction was monitored at 6-minute intervals over 4-hourly time periods. The observations made on each ward covered the period from 8 a.m. to 8 p.m. over a full 7-day week, although the 4-hourly periods did not run consecutively. Thus, for each patient a total of 840 observations was made. From an analysis of the relative frequency of interactions, one would hope to show which patients received more contact from nurses and which received less.

The quality of nurse-patient interaction was more difficult to evaluate. A system was devised whereby each patient's documented nursing care goals, which had been identified by the researcher from an evaluation of patients' nursing assessment forms, became the guidelines with which to evaluate the quality of the nurse-patient interaction being observed. Interactions were assessed and given a rating score, which ranged from 4 points if they were considered to be optimally therapeutic and in line with the stated care goal of the nursing plan (or the prescribed goal content) to a 1-point score which signified a poor nursing care outcome for the patient.

The purpose of the intermittent non-participant observation of nurse – patient interaction was to assess whether or not there was an observable and quantifiable difference between nursing action in a ward whose ward sister had a high TNF score and a ward where a low TNF score had been obtained.

## SUMMARY

The study design aimed to translate concepts identified in the theoretical framework into a range of measurement instruments to be used in the research project. The TNF indicator was developed as one method of identifying patient-centred (therapeutic) care and routine-centred (less/non-therapeutic) care performed by nurses in geriatric wards.

The study design comprised three stages. Stage 1 was linked with the construction of the TNF indicator, whereas stages 2 and 3 involved the testing and development of the indicator. The study design in stage 2 was based on a social survey approach, which involved sampling procedures and the development of a range of measurement instruments in conjunction with the TNF indicator.

**Stage 1**

Construction of the TNF indicator (theoretical perspective)

**Stage 2**

Testing the TNF indicator (social survey approach)

**Stage 3**

Developing the TNF indicator (comparative case-study approach)

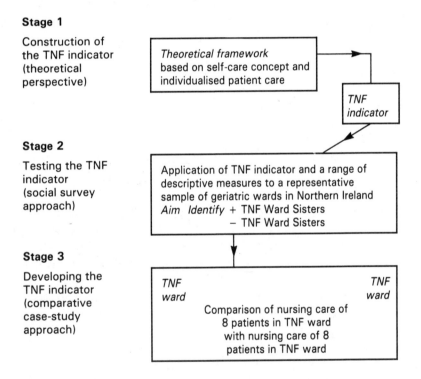

**Figure 9**  Schematic representation of study design

In contrast, stage 3 focused on two ward environments and used a comparative case-study approach to obtain more detailed and penetrating information on the nature of nurse – patient interaction, using the conceptual framework developed earlier in the TNF indicator. By varying the methodological approaches, different dimensions of the indicator were tested, the goal being to reach some measure of reliability and validity for the instrument. Figure 9 summarises the main stages of the study design, showing how the theoretical framework is the foundation on which the research is based. Chapters 5 and 6 deal with the testing and development of the indicator, providing a detailed account of the methodology and data analysis.

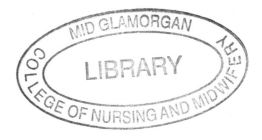

# 5 | Testing the TNF indicator

## INTRODUCTION

Having described the theoretical perspective of the study design, the aim of this chapter is to describe how these theoretical ideas were translated into reality in the ward setting. A detailed account of the social survey approach adopted to test the indicator will be given, commencing with a description of the sampling procedure, followed by consideration of the instrumentation, data collection, preparation and analysis phases, and finishing off with a discussion of the findings. The proceedings described in this chapter took place over a 12-month period, from November 1980 to November 1981, during which time the researcher was involved in full-time research.

## THE SAMPLING PROCEDURE

The focus of the study was the care of the hospitalised elderly in Northern Ireland. In defining the exact target population, however, a number of areas had to be qualified more precisely. The first consideration was whether or not it was feasible to conduct a Province-wide sample survey, given the fact that the researcher was limited in both time and resources. Two factors helped in the decision: first, very little recent information could be found regarding geriatric nursing in Northern Ireland and, second, from a practical point of view, Northern Ireland was reckoned to be a small enough geographical and demographic area to permit the researcher to consider a Province-wide project (see appendices IIIa and IIIb in Kitson, 1984).

A decision was also made to take the geriatric ward as the

sampling unit within the target population, which was defined as 'those wards that are responsible for the medical and nursing care of individuals at or over the age of 65 and who are under the medical care of a consultant physician with special responsibility for geriatric medicine'. By defining the target population in this way, a substantial number of hospitalised elderly were excluded from the sampling frame. These included elderly persons over 65 who were being treated in general medical and surgical wards, elderly patients under the care of general practitioners in GP units and those in psychogeriatric wards. The definition also excluded elderly residents in private or local authority nursing homes as well as those attending day hospitals or centres.

A sampling list was compiled by referring to government statistics on the range of facilities for the hospitalised elderly in Northern Ireland. In addition, the Chief Administrative Nursing Officer of each of the four area boards was contacted and asked to provide the most up-to-date information on the provision of ward facilities for the hospitalised elderly. Usually the researcher was referred to the District Administrative Nursing Officer (DANO) in each area, who provided information about the total number of geriatric patients and wards in the district, the name, location and size (i.e. number of patients per ward) of the wards, the designation (i.e. whether assessment, rehabilitation, continuing care or mixed) and, finally, the number of patients under the care of the consultant geriatrician. The response from the DANOs was very encouraging, and the additional information provided by them helped to update and check the information that had been collated from government statistics and other documentary sources. The complete sampling list of the target population is given in appendix IIIc of Kitson (1984).

## Method of sample selection

The sampling technique was guided by two factors: the need to ensure a representative sample and the fact that the primary sampling unit, the ward, was to provide a series of sub-sampling units including patients, nurses and ward sisters. A two-stage stratified random sampling technique was, therefore, used to obtain a representative sample of wards, patients and nursing staff. Stage 1 involved the choice of ward. Features of the ward that were taken into consideration in an attempt to ensure representativeness included geographical location, the medical policy, the age of the building, the number of patients, patient sex and designation. It was found that if wards were grouped according to geographical location, the other variables would be fairly represented in the sample. This was done by grouping wards according to their area health boards (see appendix IIIc in Kitson, 1984).

The process of selecting the stratified random sample involved writing the name of each geriatric ward on a piece of paper and putting it in a container along with the names of the other wards in that particular area board. Altogether 41 wards were grouped in the Eastern board, 18 in the Northern and Southern groups, and 19 in the Western board. The researcher then randomly selected 10 names from the Eastern board and five from each of the other area boards. This represented approximately one quarter of the geriatric ward population in the Province. (Appendix IIId in Kitson, 1984, gives the final stratified random sample of geriatric wards.)

The stratified random sample of geriatric wards then became the cluster sample for the second stage of the sampling process. Thus, the patients, nurses and ward sisters in each of the wards selected in the first stage were included as representative samples of the total population of patients and nurses in geriatric wards in Northern Ireland. The use of nurses and patients in the ward sample was considered legitimate both in terms of sampling technique and of time and resources.

A total of 25 wards was selected using the stratified random sampling technique, and all agreed to take part in the research project. Of the 639 patients included in the cluster sample, information was obtained on 631, whereas of the 343 day-duty nurses selected, information was collected from a total of 262. The relationship between the selected sample and the data-producing sample, therefore, was a close one, in that an almost total response was obtained from ward staff about patients, whereas there was a 77% response rate from nursing staff. Of the 28 ward sisters in the sample, 27 returned information.

## INSTRUMENTATION

Whereas a detailed description of the TNF indicator has already been given, little has been said about the range of instruments used in the social survey stage of the research. It had been decided to collect information on three main areas in each ward – the ward environment, patient levels of mobility and functional ability and nurse characteristics. The instruments had to collect general and descriptive information over 25 wards and within a limited time period. They also had to ensure that the collected data could be analysed comprehensively and with ease, and, where large numbers were concerned, some automatic means of coding, sorting and analysing data was preferred. Instruments that were developed included a Ward Survey Form, a Ward Profile Scale, a Patient Status Form and a Staff Questionnaire, within which was incorporated the TNF indicator.

### Ward Survey Form

The Ward Survey Form consisted of two main sections. The first section was designed to collect general descriptive data from ward sisters about their ward environment and facilities. It was based on a semi-structured interview format in which ward sisters responded to a number of factual, open-ended questions. Three main areas were covered. The introductory part gathered information on general aspects of the ward: its size, designation, age, whether or not renovations had been carried out, and information on the number and mix of nursing staff on the ward. The next part asked about ancillary services to the ward, including catering, laundry, sterile and pharmacy supplies, and paramedical coverage. The final part asked the ward sister to comment generally on her level of satisfaction with the ward layout.

The second section of the form involved the measurement of ward facilities and the assessment of ward furniture and equipment. Whereas the opinions of the ward sisters were considered to be useful in the assessing level of service provision and general contentment with the ward, a more quantitative and objective way of assessing the standard of ward facilities was preferred. For this reason, the researcher decided to measure the actual ward facilities and use these observations as a basis on which to compare wards.

Two main groups of ward facilities were considered. Patient-centred facilities included patient bed areas, toilet and bathroom facilities, day-room facilities and corridor space, whereas nurse-centred facilities included sluice space, treatment room facilities, storage space (divided into linen room space, wheelchair and equipment storage space, and general storage space), the nurses' station and kitchen facilities. A data-gathering form was constructed, with space for the researcher to note the dimensions of each facility, their number, how accessible the facility was to the main user (nurse, patient or both), how private the facility was for the patient, its suitability and whether or not sufficient storage was provided. The object of the Ward Survey Form was to ensure that each ward facility was evaluated using the same criteria. This was important in view of the fact that the researcher was expecting to come across a wide range of facilities, from old, unrenovated wards to modern, purpose-built geriatric units. Some means of classifying the range of facilities also had to be developed so that the measurements obtained could be translated into a meaningful scale that reflected the standard of the ward environment.

**Ward Profile Scale**

The construction of the data-gathering form to access ward facilities necessitated the development of a scale that would grade observations. The scale considered the range of patient- and nurse-centred facilities, outlining recommendations for minimum and maximum standards, which were based on a series of government recommendations for geriatric accommodation. Good facilities were awarded 3 points, moderate facilities 2 points and poor facilities 1 point, whereas very poor or non-existent facilities were given a zero rating. For example, in constructing a rating scale for toilet facilities, 'good' facilities had to have an area of at least 50 ft$^2$ (4.7 m$^2$), would accommodate elderly patients at all levels of dependency from chairfast patients requiring assistance to independent, ambulant patients, and were able to provide an acceptable level of privacy. Every ward had to have at least one toilet facility of this size along with smaller facilities designed more for use by semi-ambulant or independent patients. Wards that had both large and small toilet facilities were awarded top marks, wards that had toilets with an area of between 30–49 ft$^2$ (2.8–4.5 m$^2$) were awared 2 points, and wards with facilities less than 30 ft$^2$ (2.8 m$^2$) were given 1 point.

An equipment and furniture survey was also conducted on each ward visited by the researcher. Items included beds, chairs, commodes, over-bed tables, bedside lockers, wardrobes and curtaining. A brief description was made of the item, including its general dimensions and its state of repair.

## Patient Status Form

The purpose of the Patient Status Form was to provide descriptive data on the mobility limitations and functional abilities of a representative sample of geriatric patients. Demographic information was also collected, including patient age, sex, primary diagnosis and designation. A third section asked staff to identify the level of nursing assistance patients required in order to carry out certain self-care activities.

The forms were constructed so that one form per patient could be completed quickly and easily by the ward sister. Areas covered in the assessment included an evaluation of each patient's ability to move the upper limbs, trunk, lower limbs and whole body. The nurse was asked to respond to a series of specific questions in each of these areas, indicating whether mobility was present, limited or absent. A fourth column allowed the nurse to comment on particular aspects of the patient's condition. The patient's functional abilities were documented in a similar way, including activities such as washing, bathcare, feeding, dressing, toiletting and the patient's level of mental awareness. The third section of the form, in contrast, asked the nurse to indicate the patient's level of dependency rather than to identify his abilities. The dependency ratings were thought to be useful in comparing the nurse's assessment of patient ability with her assessment of the patient's dependency.

## Staff Questionnaire

The measurement instrument that was considered most appropriate in the collection of information from ward staff was the self-administered questionnaire. The basic framework of the questionnaire, in terms of orientation and question content, was developed from areas outlined by the TNF indicator. Whereas only ward sisters were required to answer all the questions relating to the TNF indicator, other members of the ward staff were asked to respond to questions related to goal content, ways of organising nursing, job satisfaction levels, problem identification and opinions on educational requirements and the concept of rehabilitation.

The questionnaire began with a series of general demographic, descriptive-type questions, which were followed by open- and closed-type questions on topics related to geriatric nursing. The decision to construct a general staff questionnaire rather than concentrate on obtaining information from ward sisters using the TNF indicator alone was made for several reasons. First, the researcher was aware of the lack of general descriptive information on nursing staff in geriatric wards. Second, having decided to study a random sample of nursing staff, it was considered politic to obtain as much information as possible from the subjects under investigation. Third, by constructing and distributing a questionnaire to all ward staff, a more detailed picture about geriatric nursing would, hopefully, emerge. This would also help to evaluate the efficacy of the TNF indicator.

The picture of the staff questionnaire, therefore, was to provide the researcher with a set of demographic and descriptive data on geriatric nursing staff. More specifically, it was to test the ward sister's performance on the TNF indicator instrument. The indicator was integrated into the questionnaire format; ward sisters only were required to respond to such questions.

## DATA COLLECTION

Before the main data collection phase began, the researcher undertook a preliminary test of the instruments in order to evaluate the content and the way in which the data were to be collected. A pre-test of the questionnaire was carried out in four geriatric wards in one geriatric hospital situated in the researcher's home town. None of the wards was included in the geriatric ward sample that had already been selected. As contact had been made with the District Administrative Nursing Officer of the area regarding the sampling list, permission to proceed with the pre-test was obtained without delay. A meeting with the Senior Nursing Officer of the hospital led to arrangements being made for six nursing staff members on four wards to be interviewed by the researcher and given the first draft of the questionnaire. The pre-test was useful in that it gave the researcher experience in arranging visits to ward areas and enabled her to evaluate the overall effect of the questionnaire design.

Following the pre-test, which was carried out in January 1981, a pilot test involving all the measurement instruments was conducted in April 1981. Three wards, not included in the main sample, were selected in another area board, and permission to carry out the pilot test was sought from the District Administrative Nursing Officer and Senior Nursing Officer of the hospital involved. The general format of each instrument appeared to be acceptable, and, again, the pilot test enabled the researcher to evaluate her own performance in collecting ward environment data and in interviewing ward sisters.

The main data collection phase commenced in June 1981 and continued into November 1981. The sample of geriatric wards had been randomly selected before the pre- and pilot tests, and once these were known, the researcher wrote to the DANOs and SNOs of the hospitals involved, requesting permission to use the ward. A brief explanation of the aims of the study was given in each letter, together with a description of the main measurement instruments (see appendix V in Kitson, 1984). The researcher also offered to explain in more detail any part of the study about which nurse managers felt unhappy. Letters of explanation were also sent to consultant geriatricians and trade union representatives.

The same procedure was used to collect data in each of the 25 wards. It began with the researcher arranging a visit to the ward in order to meet the ward sister and the nursing officer. An outline of the study was given, together with an explanation of how the information was to be collected. The ward sister was told that the researcher would have to make at least two visits to the ward; the first would involve giving the ward sister Patient Status Forms for each patient, which she would be asked to complete, and also giving her one nurse questionnaire for every day-duty member of the nursing staff appearing on the off-duty list. The ward sister was asked to distribute these questionnaires to staff, along with a covering letter of explanation, an instruction form and a brown envelope into which staff were to put the completed questionnaire and return it to the ward sister within 7 days. On her first visit, the researcher also tried to arrange an interview with the ward sister about the ward layout and ancillary services. The final activity, which was carried out either on the first visit or on the second visit when the completed Patient Status Forms and questionnaires were being collected, was the actual measuring of the ward facilities. This was done by the researcher, and involved measuring the general ward dimensions, bed area space, distance between beds, toilet, bathroom, day-room and corridor areas, and a range of nurse-centred facilities, including sluice areas, storage space, treatment room facilities, nursing station facilities and kitchen area. In addition to the actual dimensions, which were measured using a metal rule (whereas the larger areas were measured by pacing distances), the researcher noted the general standard of the physical environment and its suitability for elderly patients. A note was also made of the type, amount and suitability of equipment and furniture found in the wards.

The collection of ward facility data took between 3 and 4 hours per ward, whereas the interview with the ward sister could take between 20 minutes and 1 hour. Thus, after the initial contact with the ward sister, when the other measurement instruments were given out, the researcher either assessed the ward facilities or interviewed the ward sister. A return visit was then arranged to complete any data-gathering activities and to collect the completed patient forms and questionnaires. Although this meant a considerable amount of travelling around the Province, it was felt to be the most satisfactory way of ensuring that the patient forms and questionnaires were completed and returned to the researcher. This method of data collection did prove to be effective, in that 631 out of a possible total of 637 patient forms were returned, whereas for the nursing questionnaires there was a 77% response rate.

During the data-collection period, the researcher had the opportunity of visiting one quarter of all geriatric wards in each of the area boards in the Province, and she was able to talk to a whole range of people about geriatric nursing. The time spent on the wards measuring the facilities was also beneficial, in that the research had the chance to observe informally how nurses went about their duties. The fact that the researcher was a nurse and introduced herself as a staff nurse involved in a nursing research project appeared to encourage discussion and help ward staff feel comfortable and at ease with her.

## DATA PREPARATION

In view of the size of the patient and nursing staff samples, the amount of descriptive data collected and the fact that the researcher alone was responsible for the collection, preparation and analysis of the data, the aim was to devise a system by which some of the data could be handled by computer. Three main methods of handling data were identified, each requiring a different way of preparing data for analysis.

## Pre-coded instruments

The first method of handling data was by the use of pre-coded instruments. Examples of this type of instrument included the Patient Status Form and various questions in the nurse questionnaire, where responses were given a numerical value, using either nominal or interval scaling methods. The instruments were so designed that responses could be transferred simply onto punch cards and stored in a computer. In the Patient Status Forms, patients' ability levels were graded on a 3-point scale by nursing staff, thus facilitating easy transfer of the data to computer punch cards. Similarly, responses to general demographic information in the nurse questionnaire were pre-coded so that, when the questionnaires were returned, the information was converted into data that could be stored and analysed by computer.

## Pre-evaluative coding schedules

An alternative system of sorting data involved the construction of pre-evaluative coding schedules. Using this system, data could be categorised or given numerical ranking according to a qualitative scaling system worked out before the data were collected. Examples of this technique applied to the Ward Profile Scale and the TNF indicator.

A common feature of such coding schedules is the use of professional or government recommendations and theoretical concepts to outline the parameters used to grade the collected data. Then, by using a ranking method or any ordinal-type scale, numerical values are given to groups of characteristics that are considered to be of greater or lesser importance to the variable being measured. The Ward Profile Scale, for example, comprised a set of measures for each facility on the ward. These were assessed individually according to the pre-evaluated scale and were combined to give a composite score for the ward. Good facilities were given 3 points; moderate, 2; poor, 1; and very poor, 0.

Similarly, numerical values were given to ward sisters' responses on the TNF indicator based on a pre-evaluating coding schedule that identified features indicative of a positive therapeutic awareness (scoring 3 or 5 points) or responses relating to a lack of awareness of one's therapeutic nursing function (scoring 1 or 0).

## Classifying descriptive data

The third method of data preparation involved the sorting of open-ended responses in the questionnaire and the classification of ward sisters' responses in the semi-structured interviews. Such responses were difficult to predict and, therefore, respondents were given a high degree of freedom to say what they thought about certain topics. Although this produced a wealth of interesting and illuminating comments, coding the information into discrete and meaningful catergories was laborious and time-consuming. Examples of data that were prepared in this way include the information collected from ward sisters about ward facilities, and questions in the questionnaire that asked staff to identify problems they experienced at work and to suggest ways of improving care for the hospitalised elderly.

The preparation of data prior to analysis, therefore, involved the use of pre-coded instruments that facilitated computer analysis, the use of pre-evaluated coding schedules that classified data into ranks and ordinal-type scales and, finally, the categorisation of unstructured data into nominal scales.

## DATA ANALYSES

Two main types of data had been collected using the social survey approach – descriptive and evaluative. Descriptive data were divided into two categories. Most of the pre-coded descriptive data that were considered to be quantitative in nature were analysed using the standard SPSS computer program, which involved the use of means, standard deviations, chi squared or $T$-tests and measures of correlation. In contrast, the descriptive data, which were more qualitative were approached discursively, with little recourse to computer facilities. Analysis of evaluative data rested on the ability of the researcher to group responses into one of the pre-coded categories developed prior to the data collection stage. Observations were ranked by equating their position on the scale to a numerical value. In the case of the TNF indicator scale, these values were then computed to provide a total score. Although the numerical values of the scales could not be treated quantitatively, they identified the position of a subject on an evaluative scale by using such statistics as medians, interquartile ranges and percentiles.

## FINDINGS

It is not the object of this section to present a detailed picture of all the observations made using the survey of ward facilities, patients and nursing personnel; rather, the focus will be on attempting to describe briefly geriatric nursing in Northern Ireland and to consider ward sisters' level of therapeutic awareness. (For a fuller discussion of the results of the survey see Kitson, 1983.) The presentation of findings will be guided by considering the following question:

- What sort of environmental conditions do geriatric nurses work in?
- What kind of patient do they care for?
- What do nurses think about geriatric nursing?
- What do ward sisters think about their work with the elderly?

### The ward environment

Of the 25 wards visited, eight were purpose-built, whereas a further seven were found in old unrenovated accommodation (see appendix VIa in Kitson, 1984). The remainder of the wards – a total of 10 – had undergone some sort of renovation. Patient-centred facilities had been renovated in four wards, whereas in the other wards, both patient- and nurse-centred facilities had been renovated.

Three wards were designated as rehabilitation and assessment wards, whereas 10 wards pursued a policy of admitting both rehabilitation and continuing care patients, in a ratio of 1:3. The remainder of the wards (12) were classified as continuing care. There were three all-male geriatric wards, 12 wards with a mix of patients (3:1 ratio of female to male) and 10 wards with only female patients.

## Ward facilities

A method of comparing ward facilities had been devised by which individual ratings of named facilties could either be considered individually or computed with other facility scores to give a summary rating score. For comparative purposes, these rating scores were converted to percentages and then grouped into one of four categories. Table 1 gives a list of the categories, together with the scores and the wards that fell into each category. Appendix VIb in Kitson (1984) provides more detailed results of the individual rating of each ward facility that made up the final summary ward profile score.

**Table 1**  Ward profile scores (WPS)

| Grade | WPS score (%) | Ward | % |
|---|---|---|---|
| Very Poor | 1–19 | 11, 13, 15, 25 | 16 |
| Poor | 20–39 | 1, 2, 7, 8, 18, 20, 21, 22, 23 | 36 |
| Moderate | 40–59 | 5, 9, 10, 12, 16, 19 | 24 |
| Good | 60–79 | 3, 4, 6, 14, 17, 24 | 24 |

*Very poor facilities.*  Each of the four wards in the 'very poor' category was located in an old, unrenovated, poorly maintained hospital building, which was often physically separate from other hospital or medical facilities. Both patient- and nurse-centred facilities on these wards were below the minimum recommended standards (see appendix VIb in Kitson, 1984). Features of the ward environment included inadequate sanitary facilities for patients, inadequate sluice and waste disposal systems for nursing staff, no day-room facilities, limited bed area space with limited curtaining around beds and poor bathroom facilities that often doubled as equipment stores and sluice rooms.

*Poor facilities.*  Nine wards had an average ward profile score (WPS) of between 20 and 39%. These wards were usually located in old buildings. Four wards scored around 20–22%, whereas the remainder scored in the 30% region. Generally, wards that scored more highly in this category had been renovated at some stage, whereas the lower scoring wards had not been renovated. Examples of the effects of ward renovation are documented in

**Table 2** The effect of renovations on ward facilities in the same building

| Renovated facilities | | Renovated WPS | Unrenovated WPS |
|---|---|---|---|
| | *Ward* | *1* | *2* |
| Bathroom | | 10.00 | 0.8 |
| Clean utility | | 5.0 | 0.0 |
| Toilets* | | 3.9 | 2.5 |
| | *Ward* | *22* | *23* |
| Bed areas | | 6.6 | 5.3 |
| Bathroom | | 8.3 | 7.5 |
| Day-room | | 4.2 | 0.0 |
| Linen Store | | 5.0 | 4.2 |
| Clean utility | | 5.0 | 1.6 |
| Kitchen | | 6.6 | 1.6 |
| Toilets* | | 1.6 | 1.6 |
| | *Ward* | *7* | *8* |
| Bed areas | | 8.0 | 5.3 |
| Bathroom | | 8.3 | 5.0 |
| Corridor | | 3.3 | 2.2 |
| Linen store | | 7.5 | 0.8 |
| General store | | 7.0 | 0.0 |
| Toilets* | | 3.3 | 3.3 |

* None of the wards had attempted toilet renovations.

table 2. Wards 1 and 2 were located in the same geriatric hospital. Although both wards had an overall ward rating that was poor, the renovations to the bathroom facilities and the clean utility in ward 1 had made considerable improvements, as seen by the WPS scores. Similarly, in wards 22 and 23 in one building, and in wards 7 and 8 in another, renovations had improved the overall ward profile score. It is interesting to note, however, that none of the renovations involved the improvement of toilet facilities, which were poor or very poor in both renovated and unrenovated wards.

Although renovations improved ward facilities to some extent, they were unable to upgrade facilities from 'poor' to 'moderate' on the WPS scale. Often, renovations did not appear to tackle the major problem areas, namely poor toilet facilities, limited day-room facilities and insufficient storage space, so the wards maintained a low WPS score. One ward in this group (ward 20) had attempted to tackle the toilet problem by adding a large sanitary annexe containing several new toilets to one end of the ward. The problem, however, was that all the toilets were over the recommended 40 ft (12 m) maximum distance from any of the main patient areas. Also, the approach to the toilet facilities was made hazardous for elderly patients to negotiate because of a narrow corridor and a sharp right-angled corner. Thus, despite the extra facilities, the overall rating remained low because of the inaccessibility and unsuitability of the facilities for the elderly patients on the ward.

*Moderate facilities.*   Six wards had a WPS of between 40 and 59%, placing them in the moderate facility range. Two of these (5 and 16) were purpose-built geriatric facilities, based on the early linear design first used in the construction of purpose-built geriatric accommodation in the Northern Ireland in the early 1960s (Department of Health and Social Security, 1972 a,b). These wards typically comprised a series of six- and four-bedded ward bays, with two-bedded and single-bedded rooms. Nursing facilities, i.e. sluice and storage rooms, were located at either end of the ward, with day-room facilities usually placed at the far end. The position of the day-room and toilet facilities, in particular, was found to be unsuitable for elderly patients, and storage space was also scarce.

The other wards in this section were found in older, renovated accommodation. In terms of geriatric renovation ward standards, 9, 10, 12 and 19 appeared to be the best examples of acceptable, non-purpose-built geriatric accommodation. Wards 9, 10 and 19 shared the same basic ward layout – a central corridor divided each ward into two 16-bedded areas, with nurse-centred and sanitary facilities located between the corridor and the patient areas. Bed areas, bathroom facilities, general storage space and sluice facilities had all been improved, although toilet facilities in wards 9 and 10 were poor. Ward 12 was one of the few older buildings whose toilet facilities were moderately equipped to cope with the needs of elderly patients.

*Good facilities.*   The highest WPS scores were gained by those wards that were purpose-built for geriatric patients. Of the six wards in this category, three were examples of the later linear model of design (wards 6, 14 and 24), whereas the remaining wards were based on the more recent L-shaped model (wards 3, 4 and 17). Criticism of the linear model rested on the inadequate provision of suitable toilet facilities (generally found to be small and inaccessible to all but the most mobile of patients) and of limited day-room space. Other facilities, including bed areas, bathroom facilities, sluice and storage facilities, were good. Additional problems with the linear design were the difficulty in supervising patients in the partitioned six- and four-bedded ward bays and the distance between facilities. Day-rooms were subject to most criticism in this respect, being situated at one end of the ward and, effectively, isolated from bed areas and nursing supervision.

Those wards designed according to the L-shaped geriatric ward model showed improvements in toilet facilities and in the location and size of day-room space. Storage and bed area space on wards, and nursing station and supervision facilities, were also of a high standard.

## Patient-centred facilities

The summary rating scores of each facility were divided into five general categories (table 3). Fifty-six per cent of all toilet facilities were rated as either very poor or poor (see appendix VIb in Kitson, 1984). Day-room facilities were also poor, with 52% of all facilities being found in the very poor or poor category. In contrast, bed areas were of a much better standard in the majority of wards, with only three wards having poor bed areas. Bathroom facilities were also generally acceptable.

Good bed areas included such features as having an area of over 87 ft$^2$ (8 m$^2$), with bed centres of 8 ft (2.47 m) or more apart. There was good access to bed areas with all items of furniture and equipment, and none of the bed areas was further than 40 ft (12 m) from the nearest toilet facility. Each bed area had its own bedside

**Table 3**  Patient-centred facilities – summary scores

| Facility | Very poor 0–1.9 n | % | Poor 2.0–3.9 n | % | Moderate 4.0–5.9 n | % | Good 6.0–7.9 n | % | Very good 8.0–10.0 n | % |
|---|---|---|---|---|---|---|---|---|---|---|
| Bed area | 0 | 0 | 3 | 12 | 6 | 24 | 5 | 20 | 11 | 44 |
| Toilet | 6 | 24 | 8 | 32 | 5 | 20 | 2 | 8 | 4 | 16 |
| Bathroom | 2 | 8 | 3 | 12 | 3 | 12 | 5 | 20 | 12 | 48 |
| Day-room | 7 | 28 | 6 | 24 | 8 | 32 | 1 | 4 | 3 | 12 |
| Corridor | 4 | 16 | 9 | 36 | 8 | 32 | 4 | 16 | 0 | 0 |

locker, built-in wardrobe, cantilever table and individual bed curtaining. Bathrooms that were classified as good or very good had the following features: an area of more than 80 ft$^2$ (7.4 m$^2$) with a wide double door to improve ease of access; a free-standing bath, generally at a height of 24 in (61 cm) from the floor; and hoists also available.

In contrast, the majority of toilet, day-room and corridor facilities were rated as poor on the Ward Profile Scale. Poor toilet facilities included such features as toilet areas of less than 30 ft$^2$ (2.8 m$^2$) that were further than 40 ft (12 m) from patient areas. Door widths were also found to be narrow (less than 37 in or 94 cm) and doors inward opening. Some toilet facilities were found in sluice rooms and these along with small facilities, afforded patients little comfort or privacy. Day-room facilities that were given a poor or very poor rating were small, having less than 15 ft$^2$ (1.40 m$^2$) per patient, were more than 60 ft (18.24 m) from patient bed areas, toilets and the nurses' station, and provided little evidence of being able to offer any sort of social stimulation. Decorative conditions were also below standard, and no dining room facilities were provided. Finally, poor corridor facilities included limited area, corridors being used to store items of equipment, few visible signs or means of orientation in the ward for patients and hazards, e.g. steps or an incline, along the corridor.

## Nurse-centred facilities

Sixteen wards (64%) had sluice facilities that were classed as moderate to very good, rated in terms of location, size and provision of adequate waste disposal systems (table 4; see also appendix VIb in Kitson, 1984). In those wards with poor or very poor facilities, a major problem was lack of adequate storage space for both disposable and ordinary bedpans and urinals, along with inadequate and archaic waste disposal systems. General storage space was found to be a problem in 15 (60%) wards, a difficulty accentuated by the proliferation of disposable items. Lack of storage space was a major problem in all of the unrenovated wards, with renovated wards having only slightly better facilities.

One solution to the storage problem was to use other facilities as equipment and disposable product stores. The majority of treatment bathrooms were used in this way (wards 3, 17, 14 and 24) whereas in wards 16 and 17, certain bathroom facilities had

**Table 4** Nurse-centred facilities – summary scores

| Facility | Very poor 0–1.9 | | Poor 2.0–3.9 | | Moderate 4.0–5.9 | | Good 6.0–7.9 | | Very good 8.0–10.0 | |
|---|---|---|---|---|---|---|---|---|---|---|
| | n | % | n | % | n | % | n | % | n | % |
| Sluice | 2 | 8 | 7 | 28 | 6 | 24 | 5 | 20 | 5 | 20 |
| Storage | | | | | | | | | | |
| Linen store | 3 | 12 | 5 | 20 | 7 | 28 | 4 | 16 | 6 | 23 |
| General Store | 12 | 48 | 4 | 16 | 1 | 4 | 2 | 8 | 6 | 24 |
| Wheelchair park | 20 | 80 | 1 | 4 | 2 | 8 | 1 | 4 | 1 | 4 |
| Treatment | | | | | | | | | | |
| Clean utility | 10 | 40 | 3 | 12 | 10 | 40 | 1 | 4 | 1 | 4 |
| Treatment room | 20 | 80 | 1 | 4 | 2 | 8 | 0 | 0 | 2 | 8 |
| Nurses' station | 18 | 72 | 1 | 4 | 3 | 12 | 0 | 0 | 3 | 12 |
| Kitchen | 3 | 12 | 6 | 24 | 7 | 28 | 4 | 16 | 5 | 20 |

been taken over as stores. In other wards (5, 6, 7, 8, 9, 10 and 20), parts or the whole of the day-room were used for storing items of equipment. When treatment bathrooms that were being used as stores were discounted from treatment room facilities, four geriatric wards had functioning treatment rooms (wards 3, 4, 6 and 9). Several wards had clean utility rooms adjacent to their treatment rooms, the standard of which ranged from moderate to very good. Some wards did not have a clean utility ares, which created problems for ward staff in terms of the storing of sterile ward supplies and pharmaceutical products.

The nurses' station was a feature of purpose-built wards only. In L-shaped wards (3, 14 and 17) the nurses' station had adequate storage facilities and was suitably situated in the ward to allow access to both patient bed areas and day-room facilities. From the nurses' station, staff could supervise a total of 10 patients. In contrast, nurses' stations in the linearly-shaped wards were not adequate either in terms of storage space or in terms of accessibility to patients' bed areas and day-room facilities. From the nurses' station, a total of four patients could be observed. In the remainder of the wards, the sister's office was regarded as the nursing staff base. Here nurses received and gave reports and patients' charts and all nursing Kardex information were stored. Finally, just over one-third of kitchen facilities to be assessed were classed as poor in terms of size, location and storage capacity. Three wards, all of which were situated in old unrenovated buildings had very poor kichen facilities (3, 15 and 21).

*Ancillary services – ward sisters' comments*
The majority of ward sisters were satisfied with the catering arrangements offered on their ward. One ward sister was dissatisfied because patients' food had to be carried from the ground floor kitchens to her first floor ward as there was no lift in the building. Another ward sister had reservations about the timing of patients' meals, particularly breakfast. Most patients had a choice of menu, which ward sisters thought suitable. Meals were delivered to wards either in containers or pre-plated. Ward sisters did not appear to favour one system any more than the other.

The only problem encountered with laundry services was related to the centralised laundry system in operation in some hospitals, in which soiled linen had to travel some distance to be laundered. Problems were encountered when laundry was delayed, particularly at weekends or bank holiday times. Apart from this, the supply and laundering of bed linen and night garments was satisfactory. Personalised laundry systems also seemed to have been successfully introduced to the majority of wards. The system was reckoned to operate most effectively when responsibility for the collection, laundering and redistribution of patients' personalised clothing was delegated to one individual, either a nursing auxiliary or a domestic worker.

Problems with sterile and pharmacy supplies related to the lack of suitable ward storage space rather than to the supply of items. Most dissatisfaction, however, was voiced at the level of paramedical services to the ward. Over half the ward sisters (13) were dissatisfied with both physiotherapy and occupational therapy services, whereas 60% had reservations about the adequacy of the chiropody services. The main problems identified were the general lack of trained paramedical staff available to geriatric services and the lack of effective communication between existing paramedical staff and nursing staff on the wards. Where ward sisters were satisfied with the services, there appeared to be an adequate communication system in operation. The ward sister then felt able to make suggestions and offer advice about certain patients' rehabilitation and maintenance therapy.

Five ward sisters felt that speech therapy services were inadequate. However, the majority felt confident that if a patient required the specialist services of a speech therapist, the mechanism existed by which these services could be obtained. The opposite picture was found with regard to chiropody services.

Fifteen ward sisters felt that these services were inadequate. For those who were satisfied, either there was a direct means of contacting the chiropodist when required or a system existed whereby the chiropodist visited the ward on a regular basis – three, four or six times a week.

(For further detailed of the ward sisters comments on ancillary services see appendix VIa of Kitson, 1984.)

*Ward layout – sisters' comments*
Four ward sisters stated that, on the whole, they were satisfied with their ward facilities (wards 5, 9, 10 and 12), whereas four held particular reservations (wards 3, 14, 17 and 19). The remainder said they were dissatisfied with their ward layout. The most commonly cited areas of dissatisfaction included toilet facilities, day-room facilities and storage space. These problems were not only found in old, unrenovated or poorly renovated wards but were also criticisms of some of the purpose-built units. Ward sisters also felt that wards with over 30 patients were too large to supervise adequately (wards 1, 2, 3, 4, 6, 14, 17 and 24). They commented that a ward of between 22 and 25 patients was more acceptable, both in relation to nurse supervision and in the organisation of more individualised patient care.

Adequate supervision of patients was a problem area, which was strongly and repeatedly voiced by ward sisters in the purpose-built wards. The majority of purpose-built wards cater for up to 36 patients, and this was thought to be too many to supervise adequately. Poorly located nurses' stations and obstructive partitioning between ward bays, together with inaccessible day-rooms, were factors that were mentioned as causing problems in supervision (particularly in linearly-shaped wards). Ward sisters in L-shaped purpose-built wards also felt that ward areas were just 'too big' to supervise adequately, with the result that facilities in one section of the ward were often underused.

*Equipment and furniture*
In the 25 wards surveyed, 65% (452) of the beds were the recommended adjustable-height or King's Fund type bed. A total of 134 beds (20%) were old, fixed, non-adjustable types, with an average height of 25 in (64 cm); 10% of these fixed beds were of the old cot variety. The remaining 15% (104 beds) were Nesbitt-Evans frames, which, although in theory adjustable, were not so in

**Table 5**  Complement of chair types in 25 geriatric wards

| n | % | Description | Location |
|---|---|---|---|
| 298 | 35.2 | Geriatric mobile, backward tilting with fitted table | Day-room/bed area |
| 265 | 31.3 | Easy chair – variable back, seat, leg and arm lengths | Day-room/bed area |
| 250 | 29.5 | 193 (23%) Stacking chairs/dining chairs | Day-room/bed area |
|  |  | 57 (6%) 'Haypark' chairs | |
| 33 | 3.9 | Other types:<br>• Ejector chairs<br>• Self-propelling chairs<br>• Polystyrene 'beanbags' | |
| Total: 846 | | | |

practice because of the difficulties involved in cranking the bed up and down. (These beds were first introduced to wards in the early 1960s when many were being refurbished.)

The single most common type of chair found in the majority of wards was the mobile geriatric chair (table 5). Other chairs included easy, stacking and dining chairs. One interesting design in the stacking/dining chair category was the 'Haypark' chair. This chair had been designed specifically to meet the needs of the elderly patient and was seen as a tool to help retrain an elderly person in the skills involved in rising from a chair (Finlay, 1982). Chairs were located in the ward bays by patients' beds or in the day-room. There seemed to be an adequate number available on each ward, although one could not determine whether the chairs in used were the most suitable for each patient.

The use of cantilever (over-bed/chair) tables was widespread in the wards surveyed. A total of 455 cantilever tables was noted, accounting for 65% of all bed tables. A further 61 (8%) bed tables were of the old side-crank, over-bed table model, whereas 182 (27%) beds did not have a bed table. The majority of the bedside lockers were cabinet-type lockers, approximately 35 in (89 cm) in height with an area of 18 in$^2$ (46 cm$^2$). Eleven per cent of lockers were of the combined wardrobe-locker type and were found in three wards. Ten wards provided built-in wardrobe accommodation for patients, which was situated along the partition side of six- and four-bed ward bays. The average dimensions were 12 in × 17 in × 53 in (30 cm × 43 cm × 135 cm). Twelve wards did not provide wardrobe facilities for patients, and in such wards, patients' personal belongings were stored in communal stores, the linen store or elsewhere on the ward.

The provision of commodes and sanichairs in the wards surveyed varied from a total of nine on one 36-bed ward to one in a 33-bed continuing care ward. Andrews and Atkinson (1978) recommend that the distribution and use of commodes and sanichairs throughout the geriatric ward ought to be related directly to size, variety and standard of toilet facilities available to patients. However, the number of sanichairs per ward did not appear to vary with patient dependency nor with the standard of toilet facilities.

Results of the present furniture and equipment survey, however, compared favourably to surveys carried out by Wells (1980) and Norton (1967) (table 6).

Wells looked at the furniture and equipment in 13 wards in one hospital complex, whereas Norton obtained her data through sending a questionnaire to ward sisters in all long-term care institutions in England and Wales. Despite the different approaches, the results would suggest a general improvement in conditions, particularly in the provision of adjustable-height beds, cantilever over-bed tables and easy chairs.

Although the general impression gained from the furniture and equipment survey was one of improvement, two cautionary

**Table 6** Comparison of geriatric ward furniture and equipment from three studies

| Item | Kitson (1983) (%) | Wells (1980) (%) | Norton (1967) (%) |
|---|---|---|---|
| Adjustable-height beds | 65 | 11 | 3 |
| Cabinet lockers | 89 | 79 | 66 |
| Wardrobe-lockers/wardrobes | 52 | 11 | 24 |
| Over-bed tables | | | |
|   Cantilever model | 65 | 2.9 | – |
|   Side-crank model | 8 | 37 | – |
| Chairs | | | |
|   Geriatric model | 36 | 26 | – |
|   Easy chair | 31 | 16 | – |
|   Stacking/dining | 29 | 57 | – |
|   Other | 4 | – | – |

points must be made. First, a pattern was identified in which poor ward conditions were linked with poor furniture and equipment standards (wards 1, 2, 15, 21, 23 and 25). Here, low ward profile scores were linked to poorer bed, locker, chair and over-bed table facilities. The feeling of staff on these wards was one of having to make do with poor furniture and equipment because of poor facilities. Second, a set of quite different problems was identified in many of the purpose-built wards. Staff in wards 6, 16, 17 and 24 mentioned the dual problems of storing and maintaining a wide variety of furniture and equipment. Another problem was disposing of outmoded pieces of equipment. Frequently, such items were found taking up already valuable storage space in sluice rooms and general storage cupboards.

## Summary
The ward survey identified a range of facilities used in the care of the hospitilised elderly. Not surprisingly, wards that were found in old, unrenovated or poorly renovated buildings had the poorest standard of facilities. What is more important to highlight is the extent to which such wards are still being used to accommodate elderly, dependent patients in Northern Ireland. Over half the wards in the sample were found to have poor patient- and nurse-centred facilities, with only one-third of the wards being purpose built for geriatric patients. Although renovations had been carried out in many of the older wards, little had been done to tackle the pressing problems of inadequate toilet, day-room and storage facilities. Renovations had, however, improved patient bed areas, bathroom facilities and sluice facilities in many hospitals. Whereas purpose-built units were greatly improved in most patient and nurse facilities, problems that staff faced related to the size of the ward and the difficulties involved in adequately supervising patients because of the architectural arrangement of the facilities. Wards with over 30 patients were considered to be too large to supervise adequately, given the current staffing levels. Also, staff felt that if they were to aim to provide more patient-centred care, they could only cope with around 22–25 patients per ward.

Provision of ancillary services was found to be satisfactory in the majority of wards. Most dissatisfaction was noted in relation to paramedical coverage. Problems in this area related to the lack of regular trained paramedical staff to treat patients and difficulties in communication between nursing and paramedical staff.

## Patient profiles

An investigation of the characteristics of a cluster sample of elderly patients was carried out using a structured measurement instrument, the Patient Status Form, which was completed by the ward sister for each patient. The forms were designed to provide a general picture of each patient's mobility and functional ability levels. Emphasis was placed on an assessment of patient ability rather than disability, although the final part of the assessment tool requested information relating to the extent of the nursing assistance that patients required. General demographic information relating to patients' age, sex, diagnostic category and designation was also collected.

It was no surprise that the findings uncovered a considerable amount of immobility and limited independence in self-care skills. Geriatric patients tended to be suffering from a number of illnesses – 38% of patients had a diagnosis of multiple pathologies, whereas a considerable number had a primary diagnosis of either stroke and related conditions (14.8%) or psychological disorders including confusion and senile dementia (12.4%). When compared to results of a similar survey on geriatric patients documented by Magid and Rhys Hearn (1980), a similar pattern was found between the diagnostic groupings of the present study and those of Magid and Rhys Hearn (Table 7).

The mean age of female patients was 81 years, whereas male patients were generally younger, with a mean age of 76 years (table 8). Females outnumbered male patients by almost 3 to 1 (444 females, 187 males), and for every one rehabilitation or

**Table 7** Diagnostic categories

| Category | Kitson (1983) (%) | Migid and Rhys Hearn (1980) (%) |
|---|---|---|
| Stroke and related conditions | 19.8 | 18.9 |
| Psychological disorders | 12.4 | 16.6 |
| Arthritis | 4.6 | 6.5 |
| Heart disease | 3.0 | 3.9 |
| Diabetes | 1.6 | – |
| Respiratory disease | 1.9 | – |
| Parkinson's disease | 2.2 | 3.5 |
| Fractures | 2.4 | 3.1 |
| Multiple sclerosis | 2.2 | – |
| Other diagnoses | 12.7 | 17.8 |
| Multiple diagnoses | 38.2 | 29.7 |

**Table 8**  Age distribution of male and female patients (%)

| Age | Total | Male | Female |
|-----|-------|------|--------|
| <70 | 11.6 | 5.0 | 6.3 |
| 71–80 | 34.2 | 13.2 | 21.3 |
| 81–90 | 44.2 | 9.6 | 34.4 |
| >90 | 10.0 | 2.4 | 7.6 |

assessment patient there were three continuing care patients. The proportions of male and female patients in any of these categories, however, were found to be comparable, as were the proportions of those under and over 80 years of age. Neither patient sex nor age seemed to be a determinant of patient designation.

*Patient mobility levels*
Patient mobility activities were divided into four main descriptive categories, relating to movement of upper limbs (hand, arm and shoulder reflexes), trunk and torso mobility (sitting, leaning and twisting), lower limb mobility (leg, ankle and foot mobility) and, finally, whole body movement, which included both the ability to move and turn in bed and to change location and postural control, including balancing, walking and going up and down stairs (see appendix VIIa in Kitson, 1984). Patients' mobility levels were assessed by the ward sister at one particular time, providing the researcher with a glimpse of the general mobility restrictions and functional ability limitations of geriatric patients. The ward sister simply had to indicate whether the ability was present, limited or absent.

Generally, more patients were able to perform upper limb and torso movements than were able to perform movements related to location change and postural control (table 9). One of the few activities that over half the geriatric population was able to perform was gripping and shaking hands. This was an important ability, especially in relation to the patients' potential to perform certain self-care skills, including feeding and washing. The ability to sit upright was also present in over 60% of all patients.

The overall picture of geriatric patient mobility, however, was one of relative inability or limited ability. Just under one-third of all patients were able to move themselves in bed without help, whereas nearly 40% of patients required nursing assistance. Changes in location involving movement from the bed to a chair,

**Table 9** Patient mobility levels – summary scores

| System | Degree of mobility | | |
|---|---|---|---|
| | Present (%) | Limited (%) | Absent (%) |
| Upper limb movement | 35.3 | 42.5 | 22.1 |
| Trunk/torso mobility | 48.1 | 25.7 | 26.2 |
| Lower limb mobility | 20.9 | 42.7 | 36.4 |
| Spontaneous movement | 32.1 | 28.9 | 38.6 |
| Location change | 29.3 | 27.2 | 43.4 |
| Postural control | 17.0 | 24.2 | 58.4 |
| Whole body movement (total) | 6.5 | 32.6 | 60.9 |

one of relative inability or limited ability. Just under one-third of all patients were able to move themselves in bed without help, whereas nearly 40% of patients required nursing assistance. Changes in location involving movement from the bed to a chair, or sitting balanced at the side of the bed before transferring to a chair, were also absent in over 40% of patients, with 27% having limited ability. Postural control was similarly limited, with only 17% of patients having the ability to balance and walk unaided. These results would seem to suggest that as many as 40% of all geriatric patients were likely to be totally dependent on nursing staff for their positioning in bed or on a chair, for the maintenance of that position and for their movement to another location on the ward.

Female patients were found to have a poorer level of mobility than male patients in every activity, and the extent of these variations is shown in figures 10 and 11. Figure 10 depicts the variation in mobility and mental ability levels of male and female continuing care patients over 75 years, whereas figure 11 relates to the same criteria in rehabilitation and assessment patients. Of particular interest are the location change and postural control results. Female continuing care patients also display much greater loss of mental ability than do male patients. Rehabilitation and assessment patients, both male and female, had a greater range of mobility and better mental ability than did continuing care patients generally. It was quite clear that female continuing care patients over 75 years of age, according to the demographic information the most numerous group, were the least mobile and most mentally confused category.

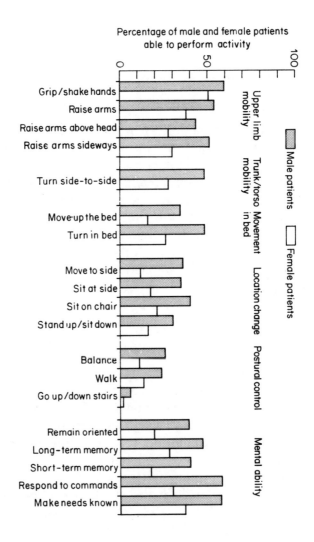

**Figure 10**   Patient mobility level and mental ability scores related to patient sex
– continuing care patients 75 years of age

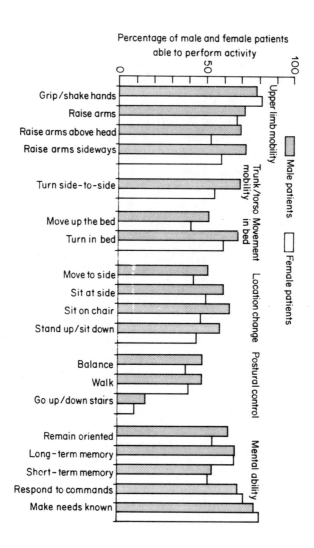

**Figure 11** Patient mobility level and mental ability scores related to patient sex
– assessment and rehabilitation patients over 75 years of age

**Table 10**  Patient functional ability levels – summary scores

| Self-care (independence in) | Degree of functional ability | | |
|---|---|---|---|
| | Present (%) | Limited (%) | Absent (%) |
| Personal self-care (washing) | 23.9 | 31.5 | 44.5 |
| Bath care | 1.7 | 11.6 | 86.7 |
| Feeding | 66.1 | 16.4 | 17.5 |
| Dressing | 13.4 | 25.5 | 61.1 |
| Toiletting | 13.4 | 33.7 | 52.9 |
| Mental ability | 28.9 | 31.9 | 39.2 |

*Patient functional ability levels*

Geriatric patients' degree of functional ability in relation to self-care skills such as washing, feeding, bathing, dressing and toiletting was also found to be considerably limited (table 10; see also appendix VIIb in Kitson, 1984). One of the few self-care activities that the majority of patients were able to perform was feeding – 66.1% of patients were able to perform this activity independently, with a further 16.4% having limited ability. In contrast, only 23.9% of all patients were able to wash independently, with 13.4% able to dress and go to the toilet independently. Male patients were consistently more able to perform self-care activities than were female patients, whereas rehabilitation patients were more independent than continuing care patients in several self-care activities.

Patients' mobility levels were correlated to their functional ability scores using the contingency coefficient ($c$) statistic. Upper limb (hand, arm and shoulder) mobility and torso mobility were found to be most strongly linked to feeding ability ($c = 0.47$ and $c = 0.49$ respectively). Ability to maintain continence was significantly linked with patients' whole body mobility levels, particularly with location change. Those patients who were most mobile were also most likely to be able to wash themselves, bath unaided and dress independently. Patients' mental ability score was significantly linked to their ability to maintain continence ($c = 0.48$). A strong correlation was also found between patients' mental ability and self-care skills, particularly in washing ($c = 0.45$) and feeding ($c = 0.43$) (table 11).

It would appear that whereas patients' mental ability is related to their ability to perform certain self-care activities, it is not as strongly associated with their mobility levels. Yet, in order to

**Table 11** Association between mobility levels and patients functional abilities (contingency coefficients)

| Mobility levels | Functional abilities | | | | | |
|---|---|---|---|---|---|---|
| | Washing | Bathing | Feeding | Dressing | Continence | Mental ability |
| Upper limb mobility | 0.45* | 0.30 | 0.47* | 0.43* | 0.40* | 0.39 |
| Trunk/torso mobility | 0.44* | 0.361 | 0.49* | 0.43* | 0.45* | 0.32 |
| Lower limb mobility | 0.47* | 0.39 | 0.43* | 0.46* | 0.48* | 0.32 |
| Location change | 0.48* | 0.46* | 0.43* | 0.54* | 0.58* | 0.30 |
| Whole body mobility | 0.58* | 0.50* | 0.41* | 0.57* | 0.53* | 0.32 |
| Mental ability | 0.45* | 0.19 | 0.42* | 0.36 | 0.48* | 1.00 |

*<0.001.

perform such activities as washing, feeding and maintenance of continence, both mental ability and a degree of mobility would seem to be necessary.

The main conclusion to be drawn from the patient mobility and functional ability scores was that up to two-thirds of patients required some measure of nursing assistance to carry out activities such as moving in bed, balancing, standing, washing, dressing and going to the toilet. Female continuing care patients appeared to be in most need of assistance, whereas rehabilitation patients tended to be more independent in mobility and self-care skills. Patients' mental ability was also found to be limited in up to two-thirds of patients, with female continuing care patients requiring more help than any other category.

## Patient dependency levels

By way of a summary assessment of patients' mobility levels and functional ability scores, ward sisters were asked to give details of each patient's level of dependency as it related to nursing activity. The areas covered included mobility, feeding, dressing and incontinence levels. It was hoped to compare the results with those from familiar studies by Wells (1980) and Magid and Rhys Hearn (1980). Although the methods of data collection differed – both Wells and Rhys Hearn collected dependency data from the same patients over several weeks – comparison of the results was thought to be useful as a means of highlighting similarities and differences between the three studies (table 12).

The results of the present study would appear to be compatible with the general trends identified by the other studies, indicating

**Table 12**  Patient dependency levels – comparative analysis

|  |  | Kitson (1983) (%) | Magid and Rhys Hearn (1980) (%) | Wells (1980) (%) |
|---|---|---|---|---|
| 1. | *Mobility* | | | |
| | Nursed completely in bed | 4.6 | 7.2 | 14.3 |
| | Nursed in chair | 37.9 | 38.0 | 48.5 |
| | Walk with help of nurse | 36.7 | 27.2 | 17.8 |
| | Ambulant | 20.8 | 27.5 | 21.0 |
| 2. | *Feeding* | | | |
| | Total help | 14.9 | 18.0 | 20.0 |
| | Partial help/supervision | 24.8 | 39.0 | 27.7 |
| | Independent | 60.3 | 43.0 | 51.3 |
| 3. | *Dressing* | | | |
| | Total help | 59.7 | 65.0 | 49.6 |
| | Partial help/supervision | 28.8 | 20.0 | 27.5 |
| | Independent | 11.5 | 15.0 | 19.6 |
| 4. | *Incontinence* | | | |
| | Any degree other than doubly | 38.2 | 36.4 | 44.5 |
| | Doubly | 27.6 | 25.7 | 24.3 |
| | Total | 65.8 | 62.1 | 68.8 |

that the level of dependency of the sample of geriatric patients in Northern Ireland hospitals is similar to that identified for other geriatric patients.

An additional area covered on the dependency form was the amount of contact that patients had with physiotherapists and occupational therapists (table 13). Over half the patients had little or no contact with either service, whereas just under one-third of all patients were in daily contact with the physiotherapist and 14.4% with the occupational therapist.

Rehabilitation patients had most contact with paramedical staff, whereas continuing care patients had least. Given the fact that continuing care patients were found to be less able in upper and lower limb mobility, posture control and body propulsion, one must ask whether or not there are sufficient resources available to allow paramedical and nursing staff to make a positive contribution to the maintenance of such patients' abilities.

*Summary*
The survey of geriatric patient characteristics uncovered a high degree of immobility and limited ability in self-care skills. Geriatric

**Table 13** Paramedical services – contact with geriatric patients

| Paramedical service | Total | Geriatric patients | | |
| --- | --- | --- | --- | --- |
| | | **Assessment** | **Rehabilitation** | **Continuing care** |
| Physiotherapist | | | | |
| Daily | 31.3 | 41.8 | 75.0 | 20.4 |
| Weekly | 14.4 | 7.2 | 10.0 | 16.4 |
| Rarely | 54.3 | 50.9 | 15.0 | 63.2 |
| Occupational therapist | | | | |
| Daily | 14.4 | 20.0 | 44.0 | 7.6 |
| Weekly | 11.3 | 9.1 | 10.0 | 11.5 |
| Rarely | 73.3 | 70.9 | 45.0 | 80.7 |

patients, typically, were female, over 80 years of age, suffering from multiple pathology and were most likely to be continuing care patients. Male patients, in contrast, were likely to be slightly younger (between 75 and 80 years old) and suffering from stroke or related conditions. Male patients, whether they were rehabilitation, assessment or continuing care, were generally more mobile than female patients. They also tended to be more mentally alert and were slightly more independent in certain self-care activities such as feeding, washing and bathing.

Over two-thirds of geriatric patients required some measure of nursing assistance, not only with ambulation but also for any movement involving location change, whether in bed, from bed to chair or from chair to commode or sanichair. A similar proportion was found to require nursing assistance with elimination, with less than one-fifth of all patients being able to use the toilet unaided. Approximately 80% of patients required assistance with dressing and 75% required assistance with washing. Up to 70% of elderly patients had limited degrees of mental ability, which put additional demands on nursing staff in terms of supervision, communication and anticipation of patients' unspoken needs. Nurses were found to receive little help from paramedical workers in the care of their patients, particularly with continuing care patients.

## Staff Questionnaire

### Demographic details
The geriatric nursing workforce comprised 47% trained nursing staff, 29% trainee staff and 24% nursing auxiliaries. There were

more student than pupil nurses in the trainee nurse section, with 70% of all students being in their first year of training. Part-time nursing staff accounted for 16% of the total workforce, with more SRNs than any other staff grade working on a part-time basis. A total of 18 male workers (7% of the workforce) was found in the sample: nine were nursing orderlies, six trainee nurses, one an SRN and two charge nurses. The majority of trained and nursing auxiliary staff lived within a 5-mile radius of their work.

Forty-one per cent of ward sisters had been working on the same ward for more than 5 years, half having worked on the same ward for more than 10 years. Nursing auxiliaries also tended to remain on the same ward for 5 years or more (30% had worked on the same ward for this length of time). In contrast, 14% of SRNs and SENs had worked for this length of time on the same ward, whereas up to one-third of trained and untrained staff had been working on the ward for 6 months or less.

Ward sisters in geriatric wards tended to be older than sisters working in general nursing areas (table 14).

Compared to Redfern (1979) and Pembrey's (1980) studies, more sisters in geriatric wards were over 50 years of age. Whereas in the acute ward situation almost half the total number of sisters were aged under 30, in geriatric wards just under one-fifth of the sisters were under 30. The modal age for sisters (W/S) was between 31 and 40, whereas for SENs it was under 25. SRNs and nursing auxilaries were more likely to be between 41 and 50 years old, with over a fifth of nursing auxiliaries (N/A) being 50 years or more (table 15).

The majority of trained staff and nursing auxiliaries were married. Over 80% of SRNs were married, 65% with children. Fifty-nine per cent of ward sisters were married, 43% having

**Table 14**  Comparison of sisters' age in general and geriatric wards

|  | Acute medical/surgical | | Geriatric |
| --- | --- | --- | --- |
|  | Redfern (1979) | Pembrey (1980) | Kitson (1983) |
| Age | (%) | (%) | (%) |
| <30 | 52 | 46 | 19 |
| 31–40 | 28 | 34 | 37 |
| 41–50 | 15 | 20 | 18 |
| >50 | 5 | 0 | 26 |

**Table 15** Age structure of geriatric ward staff

| Age | W/S (%) | SRN (%) | SEN (%) | N/A (%) |
|---|---|---|---|---|
| <25 | 11 | 28 | 55 | 16 |
| 26–30 | 7 | 8 | 16 | 8 |
| 31–40 | 37 | 17 | 17 | 24 |
| 41–50 | 19 | 33 | 10 | 27 |
| >50 | 26 | 14 | 2 | 24 |

children; of the 62% nursing auxiliaries who were married, all had children, with almost half the families comprising four or more children. A strong link was found between marital status, age of children and whether or not nurses worked part time. More SRNs worked part time, and proportionally more SRNs were married with young children.

Over two-thirds of the ward sisters had 'O' levels or equivalent (Senior Leaving Certificate) and 12% had no qualifications. Whereas Pembrey (1980) found over one-quarter of the ward sisters in general wards had 'A' levels, none of the sisters in geriatric wards had similar academic qualifications, with the exception of one ward sister who had her Diploma in Nursing. Over half the SRNs and student nurses had six or more 'O' levels, whereas over one-third of pupil nurses and SENs had up to five 'O' levels. The majority of nursing auxiliaries (67%) had no academic qualifications.

*Satisfaction with geriatric nursing*
Just over half the ward sisters had made a conscious decision to work with the hospitalised elderly, whereas 42% of SRNs and 40% of SENs had made similar decisions. Thirty-seven per cent of nursing auxiliaries said they had specifically decided to work with the elderly.

Analysis of geriatric nurses' level of job satisfaction was carried out using tools developed and used in earlier studies by Hockey (1976) and Redfern (1979). Hockey used an adaptation of Brayfield and Rothe's Job Satisfaction Index (1951), which divided respondents into three broad categories – those who had high, moderate and low job satisfaction scores respectively. The tool comprised a set of 12 statements, the graded responses of which were added together and, by assuming a normal distribution of the results of the index, were classified into high, moderate and low groupings. The cut-off points were determined by taking one standard deviation from the mean of the scores. By using this technique, Hockey found that the proportions of total hospital nursing staff with high, medium and low job satisfaction scores were 14.3%, 71.7% and 14.1% respectively.

When the results of the geriatric nurses' job satisfaction were grouped using this method, up to 90% of staff fell into the moderate range. It was decided, therefore, to use half the standard deviation value on either side of the mean as the cut-off point between low, medium and high categories. Respondents scoring between 12 and 39, out of a total of 60 points, had low job satisfaction levels; scores between 40 and 52 were moderate, and scores over 53 were classed as being indicative of a high job satisfaction level. Table 16 compares the modified geriatric ward results with Hockey's general and geriatric ward findings.

Although it is difficult to draw straight comparisons with Hockey's findings, in that the present results were obtained from a scoring system that reflected an overall change in the rating responses, it is interesting to note certain similarities. Both sets of geriatric ward responses had proportionally more high scoring nursing replies than in general wards. Staff designation and age were also found to be significantly related to job satisfaction scores at the 0.05 level. According to the index, SENs had the lowest level of job satisfaction, whereas nursing auxiliaries had highest job satisfaction scores (table 17).

Redfern's (1979, p. 178) 'intrinsic' and 'extrinsic' work factors were used to classify nurses' responses to what they found particularly enjoyable or frustrating about their work. Intrinsic factors included the ability to do things for other people, to be

**Table 16**  Job satisfaction scores

| Study | Department | Job satisfaction score | | |
| | | Low (%) | Medium (%) | High (%) |
| --- | --- | --- | --- | --- |
| Hockey | General | 12.8 | 75.4 | 11.8 |
| (1976) | Geriatric | 16.5 | 62.4 | 21.2 |
| Kitson | Geriatric | 12.2 | 56.1 | 31.7 |
| (1983) | | | | |

**Table 17** Job satisfaction levels by staff grade*

|  | Low | | Medium | | High | |
|---|---|---|---|---|---|---|
| **Staff grade** | *n* | % | *n* | % | *n* | % |
| Ward sister | 2 | 8 | 14 | 56 | 9 | 36 |
| SRN | 3 | 9 | 19 | 56 | 12 | 35 |
| SEN | 11 | 22 | 28 | 57 | 10 | 20 |
| Student nurse | 6 | 14 | 28 | 64 | 10 | 23 |
| Pupil nurse | 2 | 4 | 30 | 55 | 23 | 43 |
| Nursing auxiliary | 2 | 4 | 30 | 55 | 23 | 43 |

*$\chi^2$ = 24.42, $p<0.05$.

willing to use one's skills and abilities and to get a sense of fulfilment from the job. Extrinsic factors included areas of hospital policies and practices and working conditions. The majority of staff identified aspects of social service, i.e. being able to do things for those who are dependent, as being the most satisfactory aspect of their work (table 18). The most frustrating part of the nurses' work was related to staff shortages.

Both Hockey and Redfern identified the link between job satisfaction and skill utilisation. When skill utilisation was investigated within the geriatric nurse sample, ward sisters and SRNs were found to be most satisfied with their skill utilisation (table 19). SENs, however, felt that little use was being made of their technical, teaching and management skills. Trainee and untrained staff considered themselves to have only the most basic

**Table 18** Satisfaction with work (*N* = 196)

|  | W/S | | SRN | | SEN | | N/A | | Student | | Pupil | |
|---|---|---|---|---|---|---|---|---|---|---|---|---|
| **Response** | *n* | % | *n* | % | *n* | % | *n* | % | *n* | % | *n* | % |
| 1. Social service | 8 | 36.0 | 17 | 63.0 | 11 | 27.5 | 11 | 26.2 | 14 | 35.0 | 15 | 25.0 |
| 2. Achievement | 5 | 23.0 | 5 | 18.5 | 21 | 52.5 | 28 | 66.7 | 22 | 55.0 | 6 | 62.5 |
| 3. Ability utilisation |  |  |  |  |  |  |  |  |  |  |  |  |
|   a. Professional nursing | 5 | 23.0 | 2 | 7.4 | 2 | 5.0 | 0 | 0.0 | 1 | 2.5 | 0 | 0.0 |
|   b. Medical nursing | 4 | 18.0 | 3 | 11.1 | 6 | 15.0 | 3 | 7.1 | 3 | 7.5 | 3 | 12.5 |

Category examples:
1. 'Seeing a patient well cared for and clean.'
2. 'When I get a smile from someone who has been really ill.'
3a. 'Having the opportunity to provide physical and spiritual care, to relieve pain and to show an interest in their care.'
3b. 'To see an elderly patient being discharged who has been very ill.'

**Table 19**  Trained staff satisfaction with their degree of skill utilisation

| Skills | Ward sister | | | SRN | | | SEN | | |
|---|---|---|---|---|---|---|---|---|---|
| | Low (%) | Medium (%) | High (%) | Low (%) | Medium (%) | High (%) | Low (%) | Medium (%) | High (%) |
| Basic nursing | 4 | 4 | 92 | 6 | 11 | 83 | 4 | 2 | 94 |
| Rehabilitation | 11 | 19 | 70 | 12 | 41 | 47 | 20 | 40 | 40 |
| Communication | 4 | 7 | 89 | 9 | 21 | 70 | 21 | 19 | 60 |
| Technical | 18 | 19 | 62 | 44 | 36 | 20 | 44 | 35 | 21 |
| Teaching | 19 | 23 | 58 | 33 | 33 | 33 | 44 | 27 | 29 |
| Management | 4 | 8 | 88 | 18 | 2 | 39 | 44 | 19 | 39 |

of nursing skills but, nevertheless, seemed satisfied with their jobs.

It is difficult to explain why SENs should appear least satisfied with their skill utilisation. An additional question (45a,b) of the staff questionnaire asked staff to rank a selection of nursing grades in relation to the amount of responsibility they ought to be given in the absence of the ward sister. The variables under consideration included status of SRN, senior SEN and SEN grades in relation to length of service and whether the member of staff worked full time or part time. The responses indicated that, in the majority of cases, SRNs with less service had more authority than senior SENs with several years' experience. There was a difference in opinion as to whether a full-time senior SEN or a part-time SRN ought to be given more responsibility, 46% of replies favouring the former and 38% saying the latter. It would seem, therefore, that both length of service and full-time/part-time designation are factors secondary to the grade of worker in delegating responsibility for the ward. Although fewer staff nurses work in geriatric wards, and, of those who do, 39% work part time, the majority of staff see the SRN as having more authority than either more experienced and full-time senior SENs or SENs. These results may help to explain why over 44% of SENs felt that little use was being made of their managerial skills, compared with 18% of SRNs who felt dissatisfied.

When nurses' job satisfaction scores were related to their level of skill utilisation, a significant relationship was found between job satisfaction level and the utilisation of rehabilitation and communication skills (table 20). Use of communication skills, in

**Table 20** Skill utilisation related to job satisfaction scores

| | Nurses' job satisfaction levels | | |
|---|---|---|---|
| Satisfaction with skill utilisation | Low (%) | Medium (%) | High (%) |
| Rehabilitation* | | | |
| Little use | 33 | 15 | 18 |
| Moderate use | 40 | 20 | 7 |
| Good use | 27 | 65 | 71 |
| Communication** | | | |
| Little use | 23 | 24 | 22 |
| Moderate use | 63 | 20 | 21 |
| Good use | 13 | 46 | 56 |

\* $\chi^2 = 27.578$, $c = 0.30$
\*\* $\chi^2 = 37.259$, $c = 0.37$

particular, would seem to be linked with geriatric nurses' level of job satisfaction.

## Nurses' comments about their work
When nursing staff were asked to define geriatric nursing (part of the TNF indicator questions), the majority of ward sisters (62%) described their work in terms of caring for the whole patient, whereas 41% of SRNs and 26% of SENs described it in a similar manner (table 21). Pupil nurses also tended to describe geriatric nursing in terms of total patient care (44%), in contrast to students and nursing auxiliaries who described their work in terms of basic nursing care activities. Interestingly, 44% of SENs described their work in terms of exercising a range of personal attributes or skills, e.g. being patient, kind and sympathetic.

Nursing staff were asked to rank, in order of importance, a list of eight nursing activities that they would perform on the ward. The activities were broadly divided into routine and medically oriented nursing activities and patient-centred and rehabilitative-type activities. The most highly ranked routine-type activity was that of keeping patients clean and comfortable. Up to 44% of staff rated this activity as most important. Staff were divided on how much importance they attached to carrying out medically prescribed activities – one-third of staff ranked activities such as carrying out

**Table 21**　Definitions of geriatric nursing by staff grade (*N* = 210)

| Definition | Total (%) | W/S (%) | SRN (%) | SEN (%) | Student (%) | Pupil (%) | N/A (%) |
|---|---|---|---|---|---|---|---|
| *Basic nursing care* e.g. keeping patients clean and tidy | 32 | 19 | 22 | 30 | 38 | 33 | 42 |
| *Personal qualities* e.g. patient, kind, sympathetic | 27 | 14 | 25 | 44 | 16 | 18 | 34 |
| *Technical care* e.g. rehabilitating/giving psychological support | 8 | 5 | 13 | 0 | 19 | 4 | 9 |
| *Total patient care* e.g. meeting patients' physical, psychological and social needs in a therapeutic environment | 32 | 62 | 41 | 26 | 27 | 44 | 14 |

**Table 22**　Nursing activities of most and least importance to geriatric nursing staff

| Grade of staff | Most important nursing activity (modal value) | Least important Nursing activity (modal value) |
|---|---|---|
| Ward sister | 'Trying to create a relaxed atmosphere on the ward'　26% | 'Carrying out medical treatment prescribed by doctor'　20% |
| SRN | 'Trying to create a relaxed atmosphere on the ward'　38% | 'Carrying out medical treatment prescribed by doctor'　20% |
| SEN | 'Keeping patients clean and comfortable　28% | 'Observing and recording medical progress'　40% |
| Student nurse | 'Caring for physical needs of patient'　28% | 'Trying to create a relaxed atmosphere'　22% |
| Pupil nurse | 'Carrying out medical treatment prescribed by doctor'　27% | 'Trying to create a relaxed atmosphere'　22% |
| N/A | 'Keeping patients clean and comfortable'　28% | 'Observing and recording medical progress'　50% |

treatment prescribed by doctors to be of prime importance, whereas just one-third considered it of less importance (table 22).

The majority of nursing staff agreed that caring for incontinent patients was most time-consuming (77% of staff ranked this activity as most or second most time-consuming). Forty-seven per cent of replies ranked toiletting, commoding and toilet training patients as the next most time-consuming activity, whereas feeding patients, dressing, care of pressure areas and washing patients took up moderate amounts of nursing time. Up to 60% of staff agreed that those activities that took up least nursing time included exercising immobile patients and communicating with patients. Three categories were identified from the pattern of responses to this question: meeting patients' elimination needs was seen as most time-consuming and was, therefore, given top priority; activities that accounted for moderate amounts of nursing time related to feeding, dressing and washing; and activities relating to more therapeutic aspects of care – exercising immobile patients and communicating with patients – were found to take up least time. A similar pattern of priorities relating to personal care activities has been documented by Norwich (1980) and Rhys Hearn (1979a,b) indicating that staff will allocate time proportional to this hierarchy of needs. Thus, they found that any additonal nursing time was more likely to be employed meeting patients' elimination needs than increasing the amount of time spent exercising or communicating with patients. This observation by both Norwich and Rhys Hearn is interesting particularly in the light of a response to a question in the present survey asking staff to say what they would do if they had more time. Seventy per cent said they would like more time to communicate with patients.

In response to a set of questions asking trainee nurses and nursing auxiliaries to say how satisfied they were with reporting systems on their ward, over 60% of pupil nurses felt that they were not told what to do for patients and that not enough importance was attached to informing the ward sister about patients. Forty-three per cent of trainee and untrained staff in wards with poor or very poor facilities (WPS of less than 40) felt that the report systems were unsatisfactory, compared with 19% of staff in moderate or good facilities.

Staff were asked to identify any major problems that they encountered in their work. They were free to interpret 'nursing problems' in as broad a sense as they wished and were provided with space to note down at least three problems. Fifty-five per cent of nursing staff identified three problems, wheras 72%

**Table 23**  Problems in geriatric nursing ($N$ = 466)

| Problem | Total | | Problem 1 | |
|---|---|---|---|---|
| | *n* | % | *n* | % |
| *1. Staff problems* | | | | |
| Shortage of staff | 129 | 28 | 84 | 37 |
| Role conflict/professional conduct | 18 | 3 | 3 | 1 |
| *Total* | | 31 | | 38 |
| *2. Patient-centred problems* | | | | |
| a. Physical: incontinence | 59 | 13 | 32 | 14 |
| immobility/falls | 49 | 11 | 50 | 21 |
| pressure areas | 16 | 4 | 7 | 3 |
| nutrition/feeding | 11 | 2 | 1 | 1 |
| *Total* | | 30 | | 39 |
| b. Psychological: boredom | 36 | 8 | 10 | 4 |
| confusion | 30 | 7 | 11 | 5 |
| depression/communication | 25 | 5 | 13 | 6 |
| *Total* | | 30 | | 15 |
| *3. Organisation* | | | | |
| Nurse policies | 33 | 7 | 7 | 3 |
| *4. Environment* | | | | |
| Facilities | 8 | 2 | 4 | 2 |
| Equipment | 34 | 7 | 7 | 3 |
| *5. Other* | 18 | 3 | – | – |
| *Total* | 466 | 100 | 229 | 100 |

mentioned at least one problem; the total number of problems mentioned was 455 (table 23). Staff-centred problems emerged as the most frequently mentioned problem. Patient-centred problems fell into two main categories: physical-related problems – particularly problems with incontinence, immobility, pressure areas and nutrition; and psychological problems – boredom, confusion and depression. Few nurses perceived organisational or environmental facilities as constituting major nursing problems.

Student and pupil nurses were asked to identify certain characteristics that would make an individual a 'good geriatric nurse' (table 24). Fifty-three trainees responded, the majority being pupil nurses. Interestingly, 31% felt that the most important qualities were having a patient and quiet manner, whereas 26% saw having an understanding nature that showed kindness and compassion as most important. Only 8% mentioned some aspect of the nurse's professional skills, i.e. rehabilitation, technical or managerial skills, as being important. It would seem that trainee nurses see geriatric nursing as demanding more from them in terms of personal qualities than from a professional or technical point of view.

When asked whether or not they felt that their general nurse training had equipped them for geriatric nursing, 75% of trained nurses felt it had; only a quarter felt that improvements could be made in their training. Areas identified as requiring more training included more emphasis on psychological aspects of patient care and on patient mobilisation, diversion therapy and courses on the effect of ageing.

Up to 40% of staff indicated that they were not satisfied with the care elderly patients received in hospital (question 55, appendix IVd) and offered a variety of suggestions as to how care should be improved (table 25). Almost half the suggestions related to aspects of the nurse's interaction with her patients in terms of increased diversional and occupational therapy activities on wards, more thoughtful use of patients' relatives and voluntary workers, and increasing the amount of contact with the outside world through outings and holidays. The remaining suggestions identified areas relating to the organisation of nursing on the ward, the deployment of more staff and providing better facilities. It is interesting to note that whereas a majority of respondents noted staff shortages as a major problem (see table 23), only 4% of replies felt that conditions would be improved by employing more staff. By far the greatest number of responses identified areas of nurse–patient interaction as a key issue for improving nursing care. Improved nurse – patient interaction included more diversional and occupational therapy performed by nurses on the wards, together with increasing the amount of patient involvement with the wider

**Table 24** Requirements of a geriatric nurse – trainee nurses' comments (*N* = 53)

| Requirements | Response (%) |
|---|---|
| Patient, quiet manner | 31 |
| Understanding, kindness, compassion | 26 |
| Respect for the dignity of the individual | 12 |
| Ability to communicate | 10 |
| Sense of humour | 10 |
| Professional approach to care | 8 |
| Physical strength | 3 |

**Table 25**  Improving care in hospital – nursing staff suggestions
(no. of nurses = 105; no of replies = 422)

| | Replies | |
|---|---|---|
| **Areas of improvement** | *n* | % |
| 1. *Nurse–patient interaction* | | |
| Increase diversional/occupational therapy on ward | 82 | 19 |
| More therapeutic use of personnel – relatives and voluntary workers | 45 | 11 |
| Increase number of outings/holidays for long-stay patients | 50 | 12 |
| Increase communication | 25 | 6 |
| *Total* | 202 | 48 |
| 2. *Nurse organisation* | | |
| Emphasis on individualised nursing care | 32 | 8 |
| Establish a more homely atmosphere | 19 | 5 |
| More relaxed visiting hours | 15 | 3 |
| *Total* | 66 | 16 |
| 3. *Nursing staff* | | |
| Employ more staff | 59 | 14 |
| Improve training | 20 | 4 |
| *Total* | 79 | 18 |
| 4. *Facilities and equipment* | | |
| Better facilities | 49 | 12 |
| Better equipment | 14 | 3 |
| *Total* | 63 | 15 |
| 5. *Other* | 12 | 2 |

community through use of voluntary workers and by arranging more outings.

## Summary

Whereas analysis of the nursing questionnaire must, by necessity, be descriptive and impressionistic, a number of features were identified that were thought to influence the way nurses perceived their work. The fact that over 40% of ward sisters and 30% of nursing auxiliaries had worked on the same ward, in the same post, for over 5 years was considered to be important, particularly in relation to how nursing care was organised on the ward and how knowledge and skills in geriatric nursing had developed.

Geriatric ward sisters were found to be older than general ward sisters, and over one-fifth of ward sisters and nursing auxiliaries were over 50 years of age. Staff nurses also tended to be older, the majority being between 41 and 50 years old. The majority of staff were married with children and lived within a 5-mile radius of their work. These findings seem to suggest that nurses who would be attracted to geriatric nursing are more mature, settled and have considerable family commitments. To this extent, staff in geriatric wards might be considered as self-selecting in that, given the commonly held beliefs about geriatric nursing, staff would perhaps need some extra incentive to want to cope with a physically demanding job in conditions that are often difficult, if not impossible. What may attract this group of workers to geriatric nursing is its convenience and the personal fulfilment or feeling of satisfaction to be obtained from helping elderly people. Geriatric nurses' work was seen to revolve round the meeting of patients' physical needs and, although communication and psychological care of patients was considered to be an important aspect of care, few staff demonstrated any detailed awareness of the dimensions involved in trying to provide more communication or psychological care for patients. For example, whereas 70% of staff said they would like to spend more time communicating with their patients, few offered practical suggestions as to how this could be achieved, given the physical demands of patients and staff constraints.

Few trained staff seemed to feel the need for more training to help them in the performance of their job, leading to the conclusion that they must consider their work with the elderly as involving activities that do not require a high level of knowledge or skill utilisation. Despite the fact that a large proportion of the trained workforce was over 40 years of age, few of whom had high academic qualifications, very few felt the need for refresher courses or post-basic training courses. Student and pupil nurses, similarly, saw geriatric nursing more in terms of having the right set of personal attributes rather than having a set of professionally acquired skills.

The staff questionnaire had helped to identify the general features of a sample of nurses working in geriatric wards. In terms of the orientation of the research, however, it could do little more than point to certain responses that indicated a more patient-centred or therapeutic approach to patient care. It was the aim of the TNF indicator, therefore, to attempt to identify, within the ward sister grade of staff, those sisters who displayed a more patient-centred approach to their work and those who displayed a more routine approach to nursing.

**Table 26** Ward sisters' TNF Indicator scores

| | | | **Ward** | 1 | 1 | 2 | 3 | 3 |
|---|---|---|---|---|---|---|---|---|
| | | | **Ward sisters** | 1 | 2 | 3 | 4 | 5 |
| **TNF indicator scores** | | Maximum possible score | | | | | | |
| **Section 1** | | | | | | | | |
| Goal content | 1. Definition of geriatric nursing | 5 | | 2 | 2 | 2 | 3 | insufficient data |
| | 2. Ranking activities | 5 | | 1 | 3 | 1 | 3 | |
| | 3. Time spent | 5 | | 4 | 1 | 2 | 4 | |
| **Section 2** | | | | | | | | |
| Prescription individual patient care | a. Type of info collected | 3 | | 2 | 2 | 1 | 2 | |
| | b. Method of data collection | 3 | | 1 | 1 | 1 | 3 | |
| | c. Method of communication | 3 | | 1 | 2 | 1 | 3 | |
| | d. Information storage | 3 | | 1 | 2 | 1 | 2 | |
| | e. Access to nursing staff | 3 | | 2 | 3 | 1 | 3 | |
| | f. Use of information | 3 | | 2 | 2 | 1 | 2 | |
| | g. Problem indentification | 3 | | 1 | 1 | 1 | 3 | |
| | h. Setting time limits | 3 | | 2 | 2 | 1 | 3 | |
| | i. Monitoring patient progress | 3 | | 2 | 2 | 2 | 2 | |
| | j. Informing staff | 3 | | 2 | 2 | 1 | 3 | |
| | k. Obtaining information | 3 | | 3 | 2 | 2 | 2 | |
| Active management cycle | a. Monitoring daily needs | 3 | | 3 | 3 | 3 | 2 | |
| | b. Method of work presentation | 3 | | 1 | 2 | 1 | 2 | |
| | c. Work delegation | 3 | | 3 | 3 | 1 | 3 | |
| | d. Method of work organisation | 3 | | 2 | 1 | 1 | 3 | |
| | e. Work accountability | 3 | | 3 | 3 | 3 | 2 | |
| Survey list | 1. Nurse training | 3 | | 1 | 3 | 1 | 1 | |
| | 2. Post-basic training | 3 | | 3 | 3 | 1 | 3 | |
| | 3. Specialist areas | 3 | | 2 | 3 | 1 | 3 | |
| Skill utilisation | A. Ward choice | 3 | | 3 | 3 | 3 | 3 | |
| | 1. Basic skills | 5 | | 3 | 4 | 4 | 3 | |
| | 2. Rehabilitation | 5 | | 3 | 3 | 4 | 5 | |
| | 3. Technical | 5 | | 4 | 2 | 4 | 5 | |
| | 4. Managerial | 5 | | 4 | 3 | 4 | 3 | |
| | 5. Teaching | 5 | | 4 | 3 | 4 | 2 | |
| | 6. Communication | 5 | | 5 | 3 | 4 | 5 | |
| | B. Satisfaction with work | 5 | | 5 | 3 | 3 | 2 | |
| Rehabilitation concept | 1. Definition | 5 | | 1 | 3 | 1 | 3 | |
| | 2. Active rehabilitation | 5 | | 1 | 3 | 2 | 1 | |
| | 3. Active rehabilitation for continuing care patients | 5 | | 3 | 3 | 2 | 3 | |
| | 4. Nurse's role | 5 | | 2 | 3 | 1 | 4 | |
| *Total* | | 130 | | 82 | 84 | 66 | 98 | |

| 4 | 5 | 6 | 7 | 8 | 9 | 10 | 11 | 12 | 12 | 13 | 14 | 15 | 16 | 16 | 19 | 20 | 21 | 22 | 23 | 24 | 25 |
|---|---|---|---|---|---|----|----|----|----|----|----|----|----|----|----|----|----|----|----|----|----|
| 6 | 7 | 8 | 9 | 10 | 11 | 12 | 13 | 14 | 15 | 16 | 17 | 18 | 19 | 20 | 21 | 22 | 23 | 24 | 25 | 26 | 27 |
| 2 | 5 | 5 | 5 | 5 | 5 | 5 | 5 | i | 2 | 2 | 5 | 2 | 4 | 5 | 2 | 5 | 2 | 4 | 1 | 5 | 5 |
| 3 | 5 | 4 | 3 | 3 | 2 | 2 | 5 | n | 4 | 2 | 5 | 2 | 5 | 5 | 4 | 5 | 3 | 5 | 2 | 5 | 5 |
| 4 | 3 | 3 | 3 | 5 | 3 | 4 | 4 | s | 4 | 3 | 5 | 2 | 4 | 4 | 4 | 3 | 3 | 4 | 3 | 4 | 4 |
|   |   |   |   |   |   |   |   | u |   |   |   |   |   |   |   |   |   |   |   |   |   |
|   |   |   |   |   |   |   |   | f |   |   |   |   |   |   |   |   |   |   |   |   |   |
| 2 | 2 | 1 | 2 | 2 | 2 | 1 | 3 | f | 2 | 1 | 3 | 2 | 2 | 3 | 2 | 2 | 2 | 1 | 2 | 3 | 3 |
| 2 | 2 | 1 | 2 | 1 | 2 | 1 | 3 | i | 2 | 2 | 3 | 2 | 3 | 3 | 2 | 2 | 2 | 1 | 2 | 3 | 2 |
| 2 | 3 | 1 | 2 | 2 | 2 | 1 | 1 | c | 2 | 1 | 2 | 2 | 3 | 3 | 2 | 2 | 2 | 1 | 1 | 2 | 2 |
| 2 | 2 | 2 | 2 | 2 | 2 | 2 | 2 | i | 2 | 1 | 3 | 2 | 2 | 2 | 2 | 1 | 2 | 2 | 2 | 2 | 2 |
| 2 | 2 | 2 | 2 | 2 | 2 | 3 | 2 | e | 2 | 1 | 3 | 1 | 2 | 2 | 2 | 2 | 2 | 2 | 2 | 3 | 2 |
| 3 | 3 | 1 | 2 | 2 | 3 | 2 | 3 | n | 2 | 2 | 3 | 3 | 3 | 3 | 2 | 1 | 1 | 2 | 2 | 3 | 3 |
| 3 | 3 | 1 | 3 | 1 | 3 | 3 | 3 | t | 2 | 2 | 3 | 3 | 2 | 3 | 3 | 1 | 1 | 1 | 3 | 3 | 2 |
| 3 | 3 | 1 | 2 | 2 | 2 | 2 | 3 |   | 2 | 2 | 3 | 2 | 2 | 2 | 2 | 2 | 2 | 2 | 2 | 2 | 2 |
| 1 | 3 | 1 | 2 | 1 | 1 | 1 | 3 | d | 2 | 2 | 2 | 2 | 2 | 2 | 2 | 2 | 2 | 2 | 2 | 2 | 2 |
| 3 | 2 | 1 | 2 | 2 | 2 | 1 | 3 | a | 2 | 2 | 3 | 2 | 2 | 2 | 2 | 2 | 2 | 1 | 1 | 3 | 2 |
| 3 | 2 | 2 | 2 | 2 | 2 | 2 | 3 | t | 2 | 2 | 3 | 2 | 2 | 3 | 2 | 2 | 3 | 3 | 2 | 2 | 2 |
|   |   |   |   |   |   |   |   | a |   |   |   |   |   |   |   |   |   |   |   |   |   |
| 3 | 2 | 2 | 3 | 2 | 2 | 3 | 3 |   | 2 | 2 | 2 | 2 | 2 | 2 | 2 | 2 | 2 | 3 | 2 | 3 | 3 |
| 2 | 2 | 1 | 2 | 2 | 2 | 2 | 2 |   | 2 | 2 | 3 | 2 | 2 | 2 | 2 | 2 | 1 | 2 | 2 | 2 | 2 |
| 3 | 2 | 2 | 2 | 3 | 2 | 1 | 1 |   | 3 | 1 | 3 | 3 | 3 | 2 | 3 | 3 | 2 | 3 | 1 | 3 | 3 |
| 3 | 2 | 1 | 2 | 2 | 2 | 2 | 1 |   | 2 | 1 | 3 | 3 | 2 | 3 | 3 | 2 | 1 | 2 | 2 | 3 | 2 |
| 3 | 3 | 2 | 2 | 3 | 2 | 2 | 2 |   | 2 | 2 | 3 | 2 | 3 | 3 | 3 | 2 | 2 | 2 | 2 | 3 | 3 |
| 2 | 3 | 1 | 3 | 1 | 1 | 1 | 2 |   | 3 | 2 | 1 | 1 | 3 | 3 | 3 | 3 | 2 | 2 | 2 | 3 | 1 |
| 2 | 3 | 1 | 3 | 3 | 3 | 3 | 2 |   | 3 | 2 | 1 | 3 | 3 | 3 | 3 | 3 | 2 | 2 | 2 | 3 | 3 |
| 2 | 3 | 1 | 3 | 3 | 2 | 3 | 2 |   | 3 | 2 | 1 | 1 | 3 | 3 | 3 | 3 | 3 | 2 | 2 | 3 | 3 |
| 1 | 2 | 3 | 2 | 3 | 3 | 2 | 1 |   | 2 | 2 | 3 | 3 | 3 | 3 | 3 | 3 | 2 | 1 | 3 | 3 | 2 |
| 4 | 4 | 4 | 5 | 5 | 4 | 4 | 5 |   | 5 | 4 | 5 | 5 | 5 | 5 | 4 | 5 | 5 | 5 | 5 | 5 | 5 |
| 1 | 4 | 4 | 4 | 4 | 4 | 5 | 5 |   | 3 | 3 | 4 | 4 | 5 | 5 | 4 | 3 | 5 | 5 | 2 | 5 | 4 |
| 3 | 4 | 4 | 4 | 5 | 4 | 5 | 1 |   | 2 | 1 | 3 | 4 | 5 | 4 | 4 | 5 | 3 | 4 | 3 | 5 | 3 |
| 4 | 4 | 4 | 5 | 5 | 4 | 5 | 4 |   | 3 | 4 | 5 | 5 | 5 | 4 | 4 | 5 | 5 | 4 | 5 | 4 | 4 |
| 3 | 4 | 3 | 4 | 5 | 4 | 5 | 1 |   | 3 | 3 | 4 | 4 | 5 | 5 | 3 | 3 | 4 | 5 | 1 | 5 | 3 |
| 4 | 4 | 5 | 5 | 5 | 4 | 5 | 4 |   | 3 | 4 | 5 | 4 | 5 | 5 | 4 | 4 | 5 | 5 | 2 | 5 | 5 |
| 3 | 4 | 2 | 3 | 4 | 3 | 2 | 2 |   | 2 | 2 | 2 | 2 | 5 | 4 | 2 | 2 | 2 | 3 | 3 | 5 | 5 |
| 3 | 4 | 2 | 3 | 5 | 4 | 3 | 3 |   | 3 | 2 | 2 | 2 | 4 | 5 | 4 | 3 | 3 | 1 | 1 | 5 | 5 |
| 3 | 4 | 2 | 3 | 4 | 4 | 3 | 1 |   | 1 | 1 | 2 | 1 | 1 | 5 | 3 | 2 | 3 | 1 | 1 | 5 | 3 |
| 3 | 4 | 2 | 2 | 4 | 4 | 2 | 3 |   | 3 | 1 | 3 | 1 | 1 | 5 | 3 | 3 | 2 | 1 | 1 | 5 | 5 |
| 3 | 2 | 2 | 3 | 4 | 4 | 3 | 2 |   | 3 | 1 | 3 | 1 | 1 | 5 | 3 | 3 | 3 | 1 | 1 | 5 | 4 |
| 90 | 104 | 74 | 97 | 104 | 95 | 91 | 90 |   | 85 | 67 | 104 | 82 | 104 | 119 | 95 | 91 | 86 | 85 | 68 | 123 | 106 |

## The TNF indicator

The construction of the indicator, together with the methods used to analyse results, have been described earlier; discussion in this section, therefore, will concentrate on presenting and interpreting those results obtained from the sample ward sisters who returned the completed questionnaires. Table 26 gives a summary of the scores for each ward sister on the TNF indicator. Although representation from each ward was sought, wards 17 and 18 had no ward sister, whereas three wards each had two ward sisters (wards 1, 3 and 16), who provided information on separate questionnaires; two sisters provided insufficient data for computation of the final TNF indicator scores (ward sisters 5 and 14) and, thus, were discounted. The total number of completed TNF indicator forms, therefore, was 25.

The maximum score that could be obtained when the items in the indicator were added together was 130, whereas the minimum score was 34. Ward sisters' scores ranged from 66 to 123, and the median value was 91. Six ward sisters in the lower interquartile range had scores ranging from 66 to 82, whereas ward sisters in the upper interquartile range scored from 104 to 123 (table 27).

Interpretation of the results the TNF indicator took the form of a comparative analysis of the responses of those ward sisters in the upper quartile of the TNF scores with those ward sisters in the lower TNF quartile. Following comparison of the sisters' responses to features of the indicator, consideration was given to demographic and environmental variables that could have caused variation between the two groups.


*Comparison of high and low scoring ward sisters on TNF indicator*
Ward sisters' responses to each of the main areas of the TNF indicator were compared. Goal content was tested by a set of three questions related to the ward sister's definition of her work role and her priorities in geriatric care. The prescription phase covered two areas: questions on the extent to which individualised patient care was part of the ward policy and those on whether or not an active approach to the management of patient care had been adopted. The final set of questions covered areas related to skill utilisation, training needs and the ward sister's perception and understanding of her role in rehabilitation.

**Table 27** Ward sisters' demographic details and TNF scores

| Rank | TNF score | Ward no. | W/S | Age | Length of service | Marital status | Children | Qualifications | WPS | Patient no. | Nurse:patient ratio | Designation | sex |
|---|---|---|---|---|---|---|---|---|---|---|---|---|---|
| 1 | 66 | 2 | 3 | 50+ | 10 yrs | M | 0 | None | 22.46 | 30 | 1:2.5 | CC | F |
| 2 | 67 | 13 | 16 | 50+ | 1–2 yrs | M | 0 | None | 9.7 | 24 | 1:3.0 | CC | F |
| 3 | 68 | 23 | 25 | 21–25 | 1–2 yrs | M | 0 | 'O' levels | 21.0 | 31 | 1:2.0 | Mixed | Mixed |
| 4 | 74 | 6 | 8 | 41–50 | 5–10 yrs | S | 0 | Commercial course | 66.5 | 35 | 1:33.3 | CC | Mixed |
| 5 | 82 | 1 | 1 | 50+ | 10 yrs | M | 0 | None | 30.46 | 33 | 1:22.2 | CC | M |
| 6 | 82 | 15 | 18 | 31–40 | 10 yrs | M | 2 | Pre-nursing course | 14.0 | 25 | 1:2.5 | CC | M |
| 7 | 84 | 1 | 2 | 31–40 | 3–5 yrs | M | 2 | 'O' levels | 30.4 | 33 | 1:2.2 | CC | M |
| 8 | 85 | 21 | 23 | 41–50 | 5–10 yrs | S | 0 | IL Cert | 21.9 | 30 | 1:2.5 | Mix | F |
| 9 | 85 | 22 | 24 | 31–40 | 10 yrs | S | 0 | None | 31.1 | 16 | 1:1.7 | Mix | F |
| 10 | 85 | 12 | 15 | 31–40 | 3–5 yrs | S | 0 | 'O' levels | 45.6 | 40 | 1:2.1 | CC | M |
| 11 | 90 | 4 | 6 | 41–50 | 3–5 yrs | M | 1 | IL Cert | 76.2 | 25 | 1:1 | A/Reh | M |
| 12 | 90 | 11 | 13 | 41–50 | 7–12 mths | M | 3 | JL Cert | 15.3 | 14 | 1:1.8 | CC | F |
| 13 | 91 | 10 | 12 | 50+ | 1–2 yrs | S | 0 | SL Cert | 46.8 | 32 | 1:2.4 | Mix | F |
| 14 | 91 | 20 | 22 | 31–40 | 1–2 yrs | M | 3 | SL Cert | 33.4 | 35 | 1:2.1 | Mix | Mixed |
| 15 | 95 | 19 | 21 | 31–40 | 5–10 yrs | S | 0 | SL Cert | 46.9 | 26 | 1:3.8 | Mix | Mixed |
| 16 | 95 | 9 | 11 | 50+ | 7–12 mths | M | 2 | SL Cert | 44.2 | 32 | 1:2.0 | Mix | Mixed |
| 17 | 97 | 7 | 9 | 50+ | 10 yrs | M | 3 | IL Cert | 38.6 | 23 | 1:1.7 | CC | F |
| 18 | 98 | 3 | 4 | 26–30 | 1–6 mths | S | 0 | 'O' levels | 76.2 | 25 | 1:1 | Reh | M |
| 19 | 104 | 8 | 10 | 21–25 | 1–6 mths | S | 0 | 'O' levels | 21.6 | 20 | 1:1.7 | Mix | M |
| 20 | 104 | 5 | 7 | 31–40 | 5–10 yrs | S | 0 | 'O' levels | 53.4 | 17 | 1:1.7 | Reh | Mixed |
| 21 | 104 | 14 | 17 | 31–40 | 1–2 yrs | M | 2 | 'O' levels | 65.7 | 29 | 1:2.9 | CC | F |
| 22 | 104 | 16 | 19 | 26–30 | 7–12 mths | S | 0 | 'O' levels | 56.6 | 29 | 1:2.1 | Mix | Mixed |
| 23 | 106 | 25 | 27 | 50+ | 1–2 yrs | M | 2 | SL Cert | 16.3 | 17 | 1:2.0 | Mix | Mixed |
| 24 | 119 | 16 | 20 | 21–25 | 1–6 mths | M | 0 | 'O' levels | 56.6 | 29 | 1:2.1 | Mix | Mixed |
| 25 | 123 | 24 | 26 | 31–40 | 1–2 yrs | M | 0 | Diploma in Nursing | 60.1 | 36 | 1:2.7 | CC | F |

Lower TNF quartile

Upper TNF quartile

Marital status: M = Married, S = Single.
WPS = Ward Profile Score.
Designation: A/Reh = Assessment/rehabilitation, CC = Continuing care; Reh = rehabilitation.

*Goal content – definition of geriatric nursing*
When the responses of the ward sisters to the question asking them to define geriatric nursing were studied, marked differences were noted between the high scoring TNF group and the lower quartile. The majority of responses in the low scoring group consisted of single phrase, rather superficial responses to the question, whereas in contrast, the replies from ward sisters in the high TNF group were more detailed. Examples of the former type of response to 'Geriatric nursing is' included: 'skilled nursing care' (ward sister 3); 'total patient care' (ward sisters 16 and 8; 'really hard work, real nursing' (ward sister 18). Replies in the high TNF score included: 'involves the full nursing care of the elderly, allowing them to keep their independence for as long as possible and keeping them alert both mentally and physically' (ward sister 17); 'having a genuine caring attitude, seeing patients as individuals, being progressive enough on the ward to make alterations, to provide a therapeutic environment and to ensure patient safety without over-protection' (ward sister 20); 'assessing the patient, planning care and evaluating the success or failure of the plan ... using all resources available to the ward team to the optimal benefit of the patient' (ward sister 7). The ward sisters in the high scoring TNF group identified the importance of maintaining patients' independence, providing a therapeutic environment and being able to assess, plan and evaluate their care within a multidisciplinary team setting. None of the low scoring ward sisters, on the other hand, gave any indication of the parameters involved in caring for the elderly other than stating that it was hard work.

Ward sisters were asked to respond to two other questions in the goal content section. One area (appendix I, question 2) related to the amount of time allocated to basic nursing care activities, whereas the other area (appendix I, question 3) concerned ranking certain nursing duties in order of importance. The nursing duties that were described covered rehabilitative and patient-centred aspects of nursing care, medically related aspects of nursing and routine-type or 'traditional' nursing care aspects.

In question 2, appendix I the responses of the low scoring TNF group tended toward placing such items as feeding patients and caring for pressure areas and incontinent patients as most time-consuming, whereas the high scoring TNF group repeatedly placed toiletting, commoding and toilet training patients as the single most time-consuming activity. This variation was taken as an indication of the different priorities of the two groups, the former group concentrating on routine tasks and the latter group adopting more of 'promotion of independence' policy. This idea was further substantiated by the trends detected in the replies to question 3, related to the ranking of nursing duties in order of importance. Again, the trend in the low scoring TNF group was to place as most important actions such as caring for the physical needs of patients, keeping patients clean and comfortable and carrying out medical treatment prescribed by the doctor. In the high scoring group, the top three actions included trying to teach and encourage patients to do things for themselves, getting patients to move around and be more mobile and creating a relaxed atmosphere on the ward.

Thus, the main difference between the two groups in terms of goal content were that the low scoring TNF group defined geriatric nursing in less detailed terms and saw as important carrying out medical directions and tending to the physical needs of their patients. The high scoring TNF group, on the other hand, tended to define geriatric nursing in much more detail, outlining the range of skills required to perform the task thoroughly. They also saw as most time-consuming nursing activities that were directed towards maintaining patient independence, e.g. more time was reportedly spent commoding, toiletting and toilet training patients than was spent in caring for incontinent patients. They also saw activities such as teaching and encouraging patients to take an interest in their surroundings and creating a relaxed atmosphere on the ward as more important than caring for the physical needs of patients or following medical directives. This would indicate that this group of ward sisters saw their function as independent of both the medically dominated model of geriatric care and the traditional routine dominated model in which nursing was linked primarily to meeting patients' physical needs. Instead, the goal content of the high scoring TNF group appeared to concentrate on maintaining patient independence through a variety of nursing activities, such as providing a therapeutic environment, and by teaching, supporting and stimulating patients.

*Prescription – planning and organising nursing care*
The prescription phase covered areas such as the assessment of each patient's individual nursing needs, the formulation of

individualised nursing care plans and the carrying out of prescribed nursing action. The series of questions was based on a systematic and structured approach to nursing care planning. One possible drawback to using such a framework was that ward sisters who were more familiar with the 'jargon' of individualised nursing care planning may have responded to the series of questions in a way in which they felt they 'ought' to respond, rather than providing an accurate description of how they planned and organised their work. For example, some ward sisters noted that they used nursing care plans, stating they did so because it was the policy of the area board (ward sisters 13, 15 and 18). If this was the case, the researcher, in grading the ward sisters' responses in terms of their level of therapeutic awareness, had to look for evidence, from other replies the ward sister made, that she understood the implications of such an approach. If, therefore, the ward sister did not provide detailed and accurate descriptions of how she assessed her patients, how she collected the information and how she planned and controlled nursing care, it was assumed that she was not providing individualised nursing care, despite the fact that she said it was area policy that she had adopted. This situation meant that analysis of the prescription stage was difficult and required careful consideration and judgment of the whole information system as well as consideration of each item. In retrospect, it was felt that the series of questions might have been too intricate, and a simpler, more open-ended method of questioning in this area may have produced more definite responses. Despite this drawback, the results were felt to be a reasonable representation of the organisation system used by ward sisters to plan and implement care.

When the responses of the low and high scoring ward sisters were compared, several interesting differences were detected. The majority of ward sisters in the low scoring TNF group identified medical, social and general demographic information as important but did not refer in any detail to patients' activities of daily living requirements. There was no mention of the use of special nursing assessment forms, nor did ward sisters specify which grade of nurse was responsible for collecting such information from her patients. In contrast, ward sisters in the high scoring TNF group idenified details of activities of daily living and the patients' physical, mental and emotional states as the type of information they would collect. Although few of these ward sisters used special nursing assessment forms to collect such data, several commented on their dissatisfaction with the Kardex system, saying they would like to see a more systematic data collection form being used. Some ward sisters (20, 26 and 27) also mentioned the need to train nurses in interviewing techniques, two sisters stating that they would only permit those nurses who have been trained in such techniques to interview patients on admission to their ward.

There was more informal discussion from the high scoring TNF ward sisters about what use the information from patients was put to. One ward sister (20) stated that information collected at the assessment interview was used to plan patient care, to decide where to place the patient on the ward and to judge whether or not patients needed to be referred to other disciplines for specialist help. Another ward sister (27) noted that the information collected at this stage was not used to construct what she called formal nursing plans but, rather, that there was a system in which 'patients with problems were discussed informally and plans were made by common consent'. Generally, in the high scoring TNF group, the impression was that ward sisters knew how to use the data collected from patients, and this was linked to a more critical and objective view of the traditional nurse information system in operation. Several ward sisters commented that they found the nursing Kardex inadequate and repetitive but had to admit that they had not been able to replace it with a system that they preferred.

In contrast to this approach, the responses of the ward sisters in the low scoring TNF group did not demonstrate an awareness of the importance of the assessment interview in the planning and organising of nursing care. Several respondents mentioned medical, social work and paramedical notes as being the main source of information about patients. None of the respondents in this category mentioned the need to train nurses in interviewing techniques, nor did any indicate that they were dissatisfied with the nursing Kardex system. This apparent lack of perception of the need to obtain information about patients was further reinforced by the group's description of nursing care planning. Several mentioned the use of procedure books and additional lists of tasks that were performed on patients.

Identification of how ward sisters evaluated their nursing plans was made difficult by the lack of emergence of any clear description of the planning systems in use on the wards. Although ward sisters in the high scoring TNF group identified themselves more positively with an individualised patient care approach, few had reached a stage where they had outlined, on paper, a series of nursing objectives to be reached within a certain time limit, thereby identifying whether or not the care goal had been achieved. Ward sisters in the low scoring group neither identified problems nor evaluated nursing action, apart from ensuring that certain routine activities had been performed on all patients.

As a means of trying to identify the organisational approach adopted on the ward, sisters were asked to respond to a series of questions (appendix I, part 2, prescription) developed from Pembrey's active management cycle. The main features of the management cycle included the monitoring of patients' daily needs, prescribing and delegating work to nurses on an individual and patient-centred basis, organising work so that patients' individual needs were met and, finally, ensuring that all staff were accountable for their actions. In the high scoring TNF group, the majority of ward sisters investigated the individual needs of their patients on a daily basis by going round the patients and discussing their condition with them. Few ward sisters, however, used either individual work-sheets or nursing care plans but tended to use a mixture of the standard nursing Kardex and a variation on individual work-sheets. More ward sisters used team nursing, delegating responsibility to team leaders for the execution of the work and reporting back the results of the activity to the ward sister. Ward sisters did not appear to insist on individual nurses reporting directly back to them to account for their actions. The low scoring TNF nurses, however, tended to check only on those patients who were ill or monitored patients' progress while carrying out routine ward work. They did not see the need for a daily assessment, nor did they generally make written prescriptions of the care patients were to receive. They tended to rely more on the routine of the ward, organising their work via the staff's knowledge of the set pattern of work on the ward. Staff were usually delegated to do the work in teams, being allocated to patients according to their geographical position on the ward. Team leaders were also responsible for reporting any changes in patients' conditions back to the sister.

Although some variation between the high and low scoring

groups was detected using this method, the overall variation was not as definitive as the researcher had anticipated. No ward sister scored optimum points on every item, and some ward sisters in the low scoring TNF category were found to give replies to this set of questions that tended to contradict some of the responses they had given in the earlier section relating to individualised patient care planning. These observations led the researcher to conclude that the questions may have been too complex to determine accurately the level at which the ward sister managed her ward. Despite this, some impression of the different approaches of the two groups was gained, but, given a different method of questioning, more concrete and definitive responses might have been obtained.

The conceptual approach taken to identify ward sisters' perceptions of the prescription phase of their work was felt to be acceptable. The operational definitions and the structure of the material, particularly in relation to the active management cycle, however, were thought to be too structured to detect the range of management perspectives held by ward sisters. Consequently, in the analysis of the ward sisters' responses, the researcher had to consider each set of replies as a unit, evaluating the overall picture in terms of their consistency and looking for signs of the extent to which the ward sister had implemented the ideas in the ward situation. Comments from ward sisters relating to their dissatisfaction with the nursing Kardex system and their desire to implement more patient-centred systems were seen as signs of an individual patient care approach to nursing.

The difficulties experienced by the researcher in trying to identify distinct systems of nurse organisation were considered to be reflections of the difficulties experienced by many ward sisters over the question of managing nursing care. It was not uncommon to find wards where as many as three different reporting systems were in operation – information about patients was detailed in procedure books, in the nursing Kardex and in individualised care planning forms. Often, such situations were uncovered in wards where a decision had been made by nursing management to adopt a problem-solving approach to nursing care, but without due consideration of the specific needs of the hospitalised elderly and the nursing staff. Consequently, ward staff tended to rely on their more familiar methods of documentation, yet were obliged to complete the additional set of forms.

Although problems in the planning and organising of nursing care were detected in all ward areas, the nature of the problems encountered by the high scoring TNF group of ward sisters was quite distinct from those experienced by the low scoring group. Ward sisters in the former category generally had a better understanding of the concepts involved in the provision of individualised patient care. They noted the importance of the nursing assessment and also commented on the need to train staff in interviewing techniques and to develop more appropriate data collection forms. Many of them found the method of planning and implementing care unsatisfactory and made suggestions as to how it could be improved. The need for a more detailed and specially designed nursing care plan form was mentioned by several ward sisters. They also expressed dissatisfaction at having to revert to a task-centred approach to patient care at certain times of the day when staffing levels did not permit team nursing or patient allocation.

Problems identified by the low scoring TNF group invariably revolved around staff shortages. Patient information systems were seen as satisfactory, some ward sisters commenting that the most effective way of documenting information was by using procedure books and nursing task lists. Sisters in this groups demonstrated little awareness of the need for a detailed nursing assessment of the patient on admission, tending to rely on medical and social work notes to provide them with additional information. Individual care plans were not considered a practical reality, nor was the notion of setting care goals or reassessing the patient's individual requirements on a daily basis.

*The Ward Survey List*
Aspects of the survey list that were tested by the TNF indicator related to areas of knowledge and skill utilisation. Ward sisters were asked to rate how well their skills were being used in geriatric nursing and whether or not their general SRN training had equipped them sufficiently for geriatric care; finally, they were asked to explain what they understood by the term rehabilitation. Again, several distinct trends were noted between the high and low scoring TNF groups, which were felt to be indicative of the underlying differences between the two groups in terms of their perception of their caring function.

There was no real difference between the two groups, however, as far as work choice and skill utilisation were concerned. As many ward sisters in the low scoring TNF group had consciously chosen to work with the elderly as in the high scoring group. Ward sisters in both groups were generally agreed that their teaching and technical skills were not being fully utilised. When asked to indicate whether or not their general nurse training had equipped them for caring for the elderly, five ward sisters in the low scoring group felt that it had, compared with three ward sisters in the high scoring group. In the low scoring group, only two ward sisters felt that more post-basic training would be useful, whereas six ward sisters in the other group felt that post-basic training was essential. Areas such as the care of incontinent patients, the care of stroke patients, mobilisation and training in how to encourage patient independence were mentioned as important areas of study. Other areas included the need to retrain nurses' attitudes in the care of the elderly, the application of the nursing process to the care of the elderly and instruction in basic aspects of rehabilitation.

By having to define what she understood by the term rehabilitation, both in general and in more specific terms, it was considered that the ward sister would show her underlying orientation towards the important care goals for her patients. Did the ward sister, for example, define rehabilitation in terms of the actions of the physiotherapist or occupational therapist, or did she define it from the point of view of maximising patients' self-care potential and maintaining optimal levels of independence? Again, the responses of the high and low scoring TNF groups highlighted basic differences in orientation towards and perception of this concept. The low scoring group tended to define rehabilitation as having something to do with restoring patients to normal function and helping them to return home. Active rehabilitation programmes for rehabilitation patients involved physio- and occupational therapy, whereas for continuing care patients, rehabilitation involved maintaining independence in dressing and feeding (ward sister 3), having a homely and friendly attitude (ward sister 8), and encouraging and stimulating patients (ward sister 1). The nurse's role was seen very much as one of the supplementer of activities organised and performed by medical staff. One ward sister (16), for example, described the nurse's role in rehabilitation as 'encouraging and helping patients to do things for themselves and carrying out directions given by supporting staff'. Another ward sister described the nurse's role as being very important in rehabilitation because the nurse 'is there when the physiotherapist and occupational therapist go home'. It would appear from these observations that the low scoring TNF group of ward sisters' concept of rehabilitation was linked directly to the activities of paramedical staff. The nurse's function was, thus, important only in terms of supplementing or performing those activities normally performed by paramedical staff. Although ward sisters defined rehabilitation as helping the patient to re-enter the community or as improving the life of someone who is ill, their responses did not display any deeper awareness of how these goals could be achieved, other than through the activities of the physiotherapist and occupational therapist.

In contrast, the responses of the high scoring TNF group were more detailed, both in the general description of rehabilitation and in identifying certain aspects of the nurse's role. For example, in stating that the goal of rehabilitation was to help the patient to regain his independence, several ward sisters then went on to itemise the particular activities that would be required in order to realise this goal. These included 'restoring the patient to his former level of function, the gradual building-up of his confidence and restimulating in the patient a desire for independence, while at the same time helping him to accept those limitations that must be accepted' (ward sister 27). Ensuring that the patient is given the correct aids and equipment to achieve maximum independence was also seen as an important feature in achieving the goal of rehabilitation (ward sister 26). Rehabilitation was also said to involve the gradual reduction in the amount of aid and supervision given by staff as the patient relearns social skills and achieves a level of functioning with which safety in the home environment can be maintained with the minimum of help (ward sister 20).

Whereas the goal for rehabilitation patients was to provide sufficient stimulation to promote the patient's desire for self-care (ward sisters 20 and 26), the need for staff to recognise patients' baseline capabilities and to set realistic goals was also noted. The aim of this was to achieve optimal self-care, in which the nurse's function was to stimulate and encourage self-care activities from a realistic and informed knowledge base. Little reference was made by the high scoring TNF group to the activities performed by paramedical staff – the impression was that, in the common goal of promoting optimal self-care, the nurse's and the paramedical's work complemented each other. The focus of nursing action in providing rehabilitative care for continuing care patients rested on maintenance therapy. Here, the emphasis of the ward sister's work was on preventing deterioration and stimulating patients. Ward sisters saw the provision of a homely environment and maintaining contact with the wider community as important aspects of the rehabilitative function.

Ward sisters in this group also provided more detailed descriptions of the nurse's role in rehabilitation. One ward sister identified six role aspects of the nurse as 'one who enhances all therapy given by paramedical staff, who strives to provide an environment therapeutic to each individual, who encourages and promotes independence, who anticipates any possible deterioration in the patient's condition, who involves the patient's relatives and friends and evaluates how they can be of help and, finally, who is able to communicate with all disciplines involved in the rehabilitation process, both in hospital and after discharge' (ward sister 20). The nurse was not seen as a supplement to the paramedical staff; rather, the nurse was seen as an enabler, an encourager, an organiser of care, a teacher. Her role was also based on a firm knowledge of the limitations and abilities of the patient, enhanced by a therapeutic environment and a team of specialists. Rehabiliation was not seen by this group of ward sisters as an additional routine to be performed on patients but as a concept integral to the primary concept of providing patient-centred care, the goal of which was optimal self-care and patient independence. This compared starkly to ward sisters in the low scoring group who, whereas they defined rehabilitation as helping patients to regain their independence and to return to the community, could not define in specific terms what the nurse's contribution to this overall goal was. Invariably, they saw rehabilitation as being what the paramedical staff did, the nurse only getting involved when paramedical staff were not available.

Consideration of the skill and knowledge content of the two groups of ward sisters has highlighted a number of interesting variations. In the low scoring TNF group ward sisters appeared to be satisfied with their level of general training, the majority feeling that it was sufficient for geriatric nursing. Few felt the need for post-basic courses. Definitions of rehabilitation were vague and indistinct, reflecting an understanding of the rehabilitation process as something outside the direct orbit of nursing practice.

The opinions and attitudes of ward sisters in the high scoring group, on the other hand, were quite different. The majority felt that their general nurse training was not sufficient to equip them to care for the elderly, and several suggestions were made regarding areas of post-basic education and training. In defining rehabilitation, the ward sisters appeared to have a more detailed knowledge of the nurse's contribution to the goal of achieving optimal patient independence. The nurse was also seen as an important contributor to the rehabilitation process, acting as an enabler, encourager and co-ordinator of patient care.

Thus, despite certain constraints imposed on the data analysis by the methodology, two distinct categories emerged when the responses of ward sisters in the low scoring TNF group were compared to ward sisters in the high scoring TNF group. Ward sisters in the former group tended to define geriatric nursing in rather superficial, well-worn terms, linking it to 'just basic nursing care' and 'hard work', the physcial maintenance of patients and carrying out medical directives. Assessment of patients' needs was also sketchy, with no clear system of collecting or using patient information. Work tended to be organised on a task-orientated basis, and nursing staff were provided with information from a variety of sources, including procedure books, nursing Kardexes and nursing task lists. Finally, the ward sisters' perception of their training needs was limited, and their understanding of rehabilitation was confined to a task that was performed by paramedical staff and that did not involve nursing staff directly unless they were standing in for physiotherapists and occupational therapists.

In contrast to this picture, ward sisters in the high scoring TNF group generally defined geriatric nursing in more positive terms, identifying the range of skills and abilities required to provide a patient-centred service. Here, such activities as toilet training regimens were reported to take up more time than the more routine-type activities, and ward sisters graded activities, such as stimulating patients to take an interest in their surroundings and helping them to mobilise, as more important than the more traditional activities such as meeting patients' physical needs or carrying out medical prescriptions. A more patient-centred approach to planning nursing care was noted, with ward sisters demonstrating an awareness of the need to obtain specific information from patients and to use this in the organisation of care. The nurse's role was perceived in much broader terms, encompassing a variety of rehabilitative procedures that were not performed by the nurse by default but were her rightful domain. Ward sisters in this group also identified a number of areas in which more specialised training was required, stating that they felt their general training had not equipped them adequately to care for the elderly.

## Demographic and environmental factors

Differences in certain demographic and environmental factors between the high scoring and low scoring groups of ward sisters were noted (see table 27). Five ward sisters in the low scoring group were over 40 years of age, three being more than 50. Three had worked for more than 10 years on the same ward, one between 5 and 10 years and the others between 1 and 2 years. None of the older ward sisters had any academic qualifications, the younger ward sister in the high scoring TNF group was more than 40 years of age; two ward sisters were in their 30s and the remainder in their 20s. None of the ward sisters had worked on the same ward for more than 2 years with half having worked as ward sister on the ward for less than 1 year. Three ward sisters had up to five 'O' level passes, one had over six 'O' level passes, one had the equivalent (Senior Leaving Certificate) and one ward sister had her Diploma in Nursing (Part 1).

The ward facilities associated with each group were also found to be quite different. With one exception, the ward sisters in the low scoring group worked in facilities that had a poor or very poor ward profile score. Most of the wards had 30 or more patients, usually continuing care patients. Two wards in this group also had a nurse:patient ratio of more than 1:3. Ward profile scores of the high scoring TNF group were either moderate or good (one exception being ward 27). Only one ward had more than 30 patients and none had a staff:patient ratio of more than 1:2.9. Two wards had all continuing care designated patients, whereas the remainder had a mix of continuing care and rehabilitation patients.

It would appear from these observations that a low TNF score was more likely to be obtained from ward sisters who were older, had been in post longer, had very few or no academic qualifications and who were caring for patients in poor or very poor ward conditions. They all tended to have more than 30 patients in their wards, more patients designated as continuing care and more likelihood of having a poorer staff:patient ratio. Ward sisters in the high scoring TNF group, on the other hand, tended to be younger, had spent less time in post, had more academic qualifications, worked in better ward facilities with slightly better staff:patient ratios and had fewer patients to care for.

The development of knowledge and skills in geriatric nursing care was not apparent in wards where ward sisters had low TNF scores. This was reflected in the poorly articulated concept of their role, their poor organisational system, a limited understanding of their rehabilitation role and a lack of awareness of the need for more specialist training. This lack of skill development may, perhaps, be partially explained by consideration of the demographic information, which shows that ward sisters in the low TNF group to be older and less academically qualified and to have worked on the same ward for 5 years or more. The ward environment was not, on the whole, conducive to any kind of change or implementation of new ideas. The work-role of the ward sisters comprised keeping patients clean and tidy and coping with problems such as poor environmental conditions, high levels of patient dependency and poor staff ratios.

High scoring TNF ward sisters appeared to be more articulate, more educated and more aware of the nurse's positive and therapeutic contribution to the care of the elderly. They were younger, had been in post for a shorter time and generally worked in wards with moderate or good facilities. Their more patient-centred approach to the care of elderly people may have been encouraged by environmental factors, which made it easier for nursing staff to meet the many mobility and self-care needs of elderly patients. However, neither demographic characteristics nor ward facilities could be totally responsible for the ward sisters' level of therapeutic awareness. In the low scoring TNF group, for example, one ward sister had all the demographic characteristics of the high scoring group – she was young, had been in post for less than 2 years and had several 'O' levels, but yet had a low TNF score. On the other hand, one of the ward sisters in the high-scoring TNF group worked in very poor environmental conditions and was over 50 years of age, yet she displayed a very positive awareness of the nurse's therapeutic function in the care of the elderly. It would seem, however, to be a general finding that older ward sisters in poor ward conditions are more likely to have a low perception of their therapeutic function, whereas younger ward sisters in better ward conditions are more likely to have a more positive understanding of their role. Determining factors that are more important than these would appear to be the ward sister's understanding of her rehabilitation role, her organisational method on the ward and her perception on the training needs of herself and her staff.

The influence of medical policies on the ward sister's TNF score was difficult to assess. A broad guide to the level of contact between medical and nursing personnel was the designation of patients in the ward (see table 27). Wards were divided into three groups according to the type of medical treatment most appropriate to the majority of patients. Assessment and rehabilitation wards concentrated on the diagnosis and treatment of potentially rehabitable patients, whereas mixed rehabilitation and continuing care wards dealt with so-called remedial and irremedial patients. The usual policy in the latter wards was to ensure that 25% of patients were in the rehabilitation category, with the remaining 75% designated continuing care. The third medically designated category was the continuing care ward. Patients on such wards were those who had been jettisoned by the geriatric medical model along the path of recovery and discharge and were to spend the remainder of their lives in a geriatric ward.

Just under half the wards surveyed had a medical policy of treating a mix of rehabilitation and continuing care patients. Some consultant geriatricians seemed to prefer this method as they felt such a mix was good for staff morale, particularly that of nursing staff. With the higher patient turnover, more contact with medical and paramedical personnel and a more progressive and positive approach to care, consultants felt that nursing staff would be more able to give better quality nursing care. The influence of medical policies was, from the point of view of the medical personnel, seen to be in terms of motivating nursing staff to adopt a more poisitive and agressive approach to providing care for both rehabilitation and continuing care patients. Three wards were designated as assessment and rehabilitation wards. Each of these wards was purpose built and had been constructed to supplement already existing geriatric wards. The potentially rehabitable patients were then grouped in the new facilities close to the main hospital facilities, where medical and paramedical personnel could get on with their work. The effect of the medical policy upon nursing staff's motivation and approach to care was not directly considered: the general impression was that nurses would prefer to care for such a group of elderly patients as they were less dependent and more likely to be discharged.

The remaining wards in the sample were designated as continuing care wards. Medical and paramedical contacts were reduced in the majority of these wards; nursing staff, either explicitly or implicitly, taking over the responsibility of caring for such patients.

When ward sisters' TNF scores were related to the medical designation of their ward, some interesting trends emerged. Again, it must be stated that relating the amount of medical contact to the ward designation is but a rough guide to evaluating the impact of medical personnel. Yet is is interesting to note that the majority of ward sisters in the low scoring TNF group worked in wards designated as continuing care. In contrast, half the ward sisters in the high scoring TNF wards worked in mixed rehabilitation and continuing care wards. It would appear that the increased medical and paramedical presence in such wards may have an effect on the overall orientations and perceptions of ward sisters. It is noteworthy, however, that the ward sister with the highest TNF score (ward sister 26) worked in a 36-bedded, female, continuing care ward. Both medical and paramedical input into this ward were limited, yet the ward sister had been able to achieve a level of therapeutic awareness independent of medical policies and their positive approach to patient care.

In mixed wards, where nursing staff have more contact with medical and paramedical staff, one could argue that the ward sister's awareness of her therapeutic nursing function would be stimulated by the variety of demands that patients with such differing needs would place upon her. The ward sister would have to be more aware of her role in the rehabilitation of patients and be aware of the range of caring skills required to assist patients at different stages of their recovery process. She would also have to organise and plan her nursing care in such a way that it would take account of rehabilitation plans and social and diversional activities. The net result would be a ward sister whose approach to care would be more patient-centred by virtue of the fact that other members of the multidisciplinary team are involved in the assessment and treatment of such patients.

For the majority of sisters in continuing care wards, the medical goal of rehabilitation had long since been discarded. Sisters' views on rehabilitation were vague, their range of skills in dealing with patient problems was limited and the general atmosphere in which they worked seemed to lack any sort of positive, goal-oriented direction. However, the one notable exception to this trend, ward sister 26, was able to transfer the positive approach normally related to rehabilitation patients into a continuing care setting without the support or guidance of the medical profession. Thus, skills and attitudes that could have been attributed to the medical input into patient care required further explanation. Just as the ward sister's own understanding and perception of her therapeutic nursing function were seen to be more important than demographic and environmental conditions, so the ward sister's therapeutic awareness of her caring function was considered to be more influential in the way she provided care than was the impact of medical policy orientations. This was evidenced by the fact that the highest scoring TNF sister worked in a ward with minimal medical input.

## DISCUSSION

The results raised several questions, the main one being, why did some ward sisters provide patient-centred or therapeutic care when the majority approached their work in a routine or non-therapeutic way? Second, how effective was the TNF indicator in testing the therapeutic awareness of ward sisters? Finally, what effect did the high scoring TNF ward sisters have on other members of nursing staff and on the quality of patient care?

Both Baker (1978) and Evers (1981b) identified two groups of workers in geriatric nursing care. The larger group comprised routine-oriented nursing personnel, whose attitudes and perceptions about care of the hospitalised elderly were seen to reflect a medically dominated approach to care or a custodial model. Either way, the result was the same: staff viewed elderly patients who did not conform to the medical model goals of assessment, diagnosis, treatment and cure as failures, whereas in the custodial model ethos, patients were seen as social failures. However, Baker and Evers differed somewhat in their explanation of why a minority of nurses chose to provide more patient-centred care. Evers believed that ward sisters gave this type of care when they had delegated responsibility for the care of continuing care patients and when the implicit definition of the care task was seen as valid in its own right. She felt that this situation was related to the structure of social relations among members of multi-disciplinary care team and, most importantly, between ward sisters and consultant geriatricians. She saw the working relationship between doctors and nurses as crucial in relation to whether long-stay care work was defined as a valid and valuable alternative to cure work or whether it was seen merely as a result of a failure of the medical strategy.

Whereas Baker (1978) acknowledged the influence of the medical model, interrelated with a range of organisational and social factors, she felt that ward sisters' beliefs about nursing ought to be considered in attempting to explain why a minority chose to provide patient-centred care. She identified as particularly important the nurse's perception of her caring role in the provision of such care, and called for the re-ordering of priorities that would accept the nurse's caring role as fundamental to nursing. Baker's comments serve to underline the importance of the issues under investigation in the present study, namely that geriatric nursing's main problem is that it lacks a theoretical framework on which to build its concepts of care. In consequence, nursing care on the wards is influenced by a variety of external factors, whether they be poor ward facilities, cure-oriented medical policies or a custodial model of care inherited from the Poor Law. The argument is that the difference between therapeutic and non-therapeutic, or patient-centred and routine-centred, ward sisters is that the former group provide better care because they have accepted care as their central role. This concept of care was given substance through the theoretical framework developed for geriatric care and the TNF indicator. How effective the TNF indicator was in testing the beliefs and orientations of wards sisters will be considered in chapter 6. This will be attempted by looking at each of the items on the TNF indicator and relating them to the actual ward situation, where the goal is to provide patient-centred care.

# 6 Developing the TNF indicator

## INTRODUCTION

The nurse's, or more specifically, the ward sister's therapeutic nursing function has been identified as involving a particular conceptual approach to the care of the elderly. It also involves an organisational approach based on patient-centred care, an active management cycle for delegating work on the ward, and an awareness of the range of skills and knowledge required to provide care for the hospitalised elderly. This therapeutic awareness is more likely to be found in ward sisters who are younger, who have been in post for less than 2 years, who have more academic qualifications, who work in wards with a mix of rehabilitation and continuing care patients, and where the ward facilities are moderate to good.

An important feature of the nurse's therapeutic function is her perception of her caring role. Nursing action is considered therapeutic only if it combines a patient-centred system of care with a range of personal and emotional aspects. Thus, the ward sister who displays a therapeutic approach to care would not only organise and delegate her work in a particular way, but would also communicate and deal with patients on a more personal level. This would involve consciously making use of her personality to encourage or help a patient, becoming more involved in personal exchanges with patients and recognising the need to respond, to feel and to provide comfort for patients.

Where the testing of the TNF indicator identified the main organisational components, the more personal elements of the nurse's caring role were not as clearly documented. These aspects were thought to be observed most effectively in the natural ward setting, where nurses and patients are involved in daily interactions.

155

In addition to providing information on the more interpersonal aspects of nurse–patient interaction, a detailed study of two ward environments was undertaken to test whether or not the ward sister's TNF score affected the quantity and quality of care provided to patients. It was argued that ward sisters with a high TNF score were more likely to demonstrate a more personal and sensitive approach to patient care and to organise nursing care in a more patient-centred way than were low scoring TNF ward sisters. The aim of this final study, therefore, was to investigate whether the quantity and quality of nursing care was better in a ward whose sister had a high TNF score than in a ward where the sister had a low TNF score.

## THE CASE-STUDY APPROACH

Because of the interpersonal nature of the characteristics under scrutiny, the most appropriate method of investigation was felt to be the case-study approach. Abdellah and Levine (1979) have described it as a 'detailed, factual, largely narrative description and analysis of institutions ... or group of individuals in their natural setting'. They state (p.56) that the case study may include statistical data as well as verbal descriptions, together with explanatory and evaluative statements. Fox (1982) notes that the case-study approach is used when seeking depth of information, which cannot usually be obtained from a large number of respondents. Thus, whereas the social survey approach had been able to identify general trends and opinions of ward sisters' therapeutic awareness, the case study was to focus on the experiences of several patients in contrasting ward environments in order to evaluate the quality of nursing care they were receiving.

### Choice of ward

The social survey approach had shown that a number of extraneous variables were linked to the ward sister's TNF score. In the case study, an attempt was made to control as many of these variables as possible. These included the standard of ward facilities, and medical, paramedical and nurse management constraints. A simple way of doing this was to compare the nursing care on two wards in the same geriatric unit, the main variation being the ward sisters' TNF score. A further determinant in the choice of wards was their accessibility to the researcher, i.e. they needed to be convenient for the several weeks of observational study that would be undertaken. As it happened, two wards in the high TNF quartile (wards 24 and 25) were within a 5-mile radius of the researcher's home. Ward 24 was chosen as the more appropriate ward for the case study. Its ward sister had the highest TNF score and its ward facilities were graded as moderate. The ward was located in the upper floor of a two-ward geriatric unit that had been built in the grounds of the local hospital in the early 1970s to replace other geriatric accommodation. A physiotherapy and occupational therapy department was also attached to the geriatric unit. The facilities on ward 24 and the lower ward in the unit were similar, as was involvement from medical and paramedical staff. One nursing officer was responsible for the wards, together with two other geriatric wards located in another part of the hospital complex.

It was decided to use ward 24 (hereafter called 'White Ward') and its adjacent ward (hereafter called 'Brown Ward') in the study, but, before this, the researcher had to determine the TNF score of the ward sister in Brown Ward as it had not been involved in the social survey. The nursing officer was approached and a request made to the ward sister to complete one of the staff questionnaires in which were contained the TNF indicator questions. The ward sister was found to have a TNF score of 83 (see appendix III). Although just outside the lower interquartile range, this score was considered to be sufficiently distinct from that of the ward sister in ward 24, who had a score of 123, to allow the study to proceed.

To test further the relative influence on patient care of the ward sister and environmental or medical policies, it was decided to extend the comparative analysis to include the study of nursing on a third ward ('Red Ward'). Red ward was distinguished by its progressive medical and paramedical approach to geriatric care and its high standard of ward facilities, yet the ward sister's TNF score was found to be in the lower interquartile range (see appendix III). The researcher was interested to see how the ward sister's behaviour compared with that of the high scoring TNF sister in White Ward and the low scoring TNF sister in Brown Ward. In addition, it would be interesting to observe how the different medical, paramedical and ward facilities affected the quantity and quality of nursing.

## The role of the researcher

Because of the more detailed approach to data gathering, which is a characteristic of case studies, the researcher's role in the data-gathering phase changed from that of a rather unobtrusive figure in the ward to a much more closely involved one. Over a period stretching from May 1982 to December 1982, the researcher became the main data gatherer, observing and contrasting patient care and nursing action in three different geriatric ward environments. In order to minimise the potentially disruptive effect that her presence could have had on the normal work pattern of the ward, the researcher adopted the following techniques for carrying out observations: first, she circulated an information sheet to nursing staff in the ward, explaining in general terms what the study was about and how long it would continue; second, she stressed that observations would focus on *patient* action and responses rather than on nursing activity; third, only when nurses interacted with those patients whom the researcher was observing, would the nurse's activity be noted. It was felt that by emphasising the researcher's primary interest in patients' experiences, staff would feel less threatened and would, therefore, act in a more relaxed and normal manner. In order to be as unobtrusive as possible to patients, the researcher chose to study in detail the activities of eight patients who were located throughout the ward. This meant that the researcher was constantly moving about and not ostensibly 'spying' on any particular patient group. The patients who were chosen were selected as representative of the most common type of patient in geriatric wards (see appendix VIIIc in Kitson, 1984). They were matched for levels of mobility and functional ability and grouped into one of three main nursing systems (see table 28, page 165). Another safeguard in trying to ensure as normal a behaviour as possible was that neither staff nor patients were told which patients were being observed.

A final technique adopted by the researcher to help in the comparative case study related to the methods by which incidents were observed and documented. It involved extensive use of the geriatric nursing theoretical framework developed earlier to guide and direct the way in which interactions were quantified and, more importantly, the way in which they were evaluated.

## METHODOLOGY

The effect of nursing action on patient outcomes could be assessed both quantitatively and qualitatively. From the quantitative point of view, the frequency and duration of activities in one ward could be compared with similar activities on the other wards. This would require an observation schedule that would note the type, frequency and duration of the activity. A more complex set of observational guidelines would be needed to determine the quality of patient activity. This was seen to require the development of a scale that would grade particular acts in areas of patient self-care in terms of each action's therapeutic content. Therapeutic nursing activity, which was seen as a precursor to therapeutic outcomes of patient care, was determined from the geriatric nursing theoretical framework based on the concept of optimal self-care as the primary goal of nursing care.

### Quantitative data

An intermittent, non-participant observation technique was used to collect data relating to patient and nurse activity on the ward. Work study analyses have found that intermittent observations on a regular, pre-set time interval present accurate pictures of the overall situation under scrutiny (Whitmore, 1970). The basis of such studies is that a sample taken at random from a small group tends to have the same pattern of distribution as the larger group. The time interval between observations is often determined by the nature of the activity being observed. In repetitive-type jobs, where the activity is easily recognisable and recurs frequently, time intervals are short – between 2 and 3 minutes. Observation of nursing activity, however, needs to provide the observer with sufficient time to be able to assess the activity, which may be one of a number of distinct actions. The same situation occurs with observation of patient activity, with or without nursing assistance. The time interval between observations, consequently, is often around 5 or 6 minutes. The method of data collection and the number of subjects being observed will also effect the time interval chosen. During the first few days on the ward, the researcher tested the amount of information she could collect from patients within particular time limits. It was found that adequate notes on the activities of eight patients could be made within 6-minute intervals.

*The observation schedule (appendix IV)*

The observation schedule had to ensure that information was collected on both the frequency and the quality of patient and nurse action. Consequently, a system was devised in which the observations were written down in long-hand by the researcher as they occurred on the ward. Each interaction between the patient and the nurse was observed up to the point at which the researcher could describe it in a detailed and meaningful way. In the same way, patient activity that was not performed with nursing assistance was noted and observed up to a point within each 6-minute cycle at which the researcher could describe the action in a meaningful way. General patterns of ward activity were also noted on the observation schedule. For example, staff break times and shift changing times were noted as these affected the number of nurses on the ward. A 6-minute observation cycle was maintained and was found to accommodate the variations in the length of time required by the researcher to document fully the activities taking place. As the patients being observed were scattered throughout the ward, patients at one end of the ward would often be involved in certain self-care activities with nurses whereas patients at the other end would not be involved in any sort of activity. Thus, whereas the time taken to observe the interactions of certain patients with nurses could be up to 1 or 1½ minutes, other patient activities could be judged at a glance.

One problem area was when patients were out of the direct view of the researcher, for example, when they were behind curtains or a closed door. The researcher had to decide whether she was going to invade patients' privacy during certain procedures and jeopardise their anonymity or risk losing important observations on nurse–patient activity. Somewhat serendipitously, the problem was resolved by the fact that several of the nursing staff were not consistent in pulling curtains completely round patients while performing certain activities, which thus provided the researcher with the opportunity of observing these more intimate interactions. The problem of closed doors was also minimised by the fact that very few nurses chose to close toilet doors or leave patients unattended and out of sight. The main problem area was when patients were bathed. The researcher did not follow patients into the bathroom and was, therefore, unable to obtain any sort of qualitative information about the way the activity was carried out by staff. When patients left the ward to go to physiotherapy and occupational therapy, the researcher followed, maintaining the 6-minute interval. Approximately half the patients being observed in each of the wards attended physiotherapy, occupational therapy or some other sort of activity outside the ward. This meant that for certain periods the number of patients being observed on the ward was reduced by 50%.

A total of 10 observations was recorded per hour. The researcher remained on the ward for 4 hours at a time, thus dividing the observations into morning, afternoon and evening periods (8 a.m. to 12 noon, 12 noon to 4 p.m. and 4 p.m. to 8 p.m. respectively). Each day of the week was covered, from 8 a.m. until 8 p.m., resulting in a total of 840 ($10 \times 12 \times 7$) observations per patient. No more than one observation period was conducted on any day, thus requiring 21 separate days for ward observations. The researcher spent between 6 and 8 weeks on each ward to obtain the full set of observations.

## Coding the observations (see appendixes V and VI)

Given the number of observations per patient (840) and the number of patients per ward (8), the method of coding the observations had to take account of the need to analyse data by computer. This led to the development of a coding list which gave a numerical value to each type of activity observed (see appendix V). The activities were divided into three main areas. The first comprised basic self-care activities, such as elimination, feeding, drinking, washing, bathing, dressing, undressing, exercising and communication. The next category was contact with other workers – doctors, paramedical workers (particularly the physiotherapist and occupational therapist) and other personnel, such as hairdressers, art therapists and chiropodists. Visitors were also included in this group, together with ministers of religion and voluntary workers. The third section dealt with the location of the patient in the ward.

The observations for each patient were transferred from the original observation schedule to a series of coding forms, which provided five units of space in which to describe the nursing activities (see appendix VI). Each coding frame contained 12 hours of observations, and each patient had seven such forms. Reading the five-unit columns from left to right, the first two units contained the activity code, whereas the other three units described the quality of the self-care activity. Zero scores were

recorded in these boxes when the patient was inactive. These data
were then ready for computer analysis. The SPSS program was
used both to provide quantitative data, in the form of frequency
distributions on the time spent on certain activities, and to
determine whether or not any differences could be detected
between the amount of time that patients spent in certain activities
in Brown Ward compared to White Ward and, later, Red ward
compared to Brown Ward.

## Qualitative data

Several methods have been used to evaluate quality of nursing
care. One way is to link quality with quantity, arguing that if an
activity has been performed a number of times, it guarantees a
certain level of quality of care (Adams and McIlwraith, 1963;
Scottish Home and Health Department, 1967). More recent
studies have related the number of times the activity has been
performed to the outcome (British Geriatric Society and Royal
College of Nursing, 1975; Rhys Hearn, 1979 a,b). However, the
question still remains as to what one measures quality of care
against. Linking nursing outcomes with prescribed nursing care
would seem to be one area of possible development in the search
for a quality indicator (Bloch, 1975; Luker, 1981). With this
approach, the nurse needs to be able to assess patients' individual
needs, plan care and evaluate the outcome, and to do this in such
a way that patients' dignity and independence are maintained.

It is argued that before nurses can give individualised care that
has as its goal optimal self-care and independence for each patient,
they must come to a point where they view themselves and their
activities in a positive and dynamic way. In observing the quality
of nurse–patient interaction in the geriatric ward setting, aspects
of the nurse's activity that would indicate a therapeutic or
dynamic approach would include her awareness of the capabilities
(or self-care approach) of the patient, her ability to provide
sufficient help and support for the patient without taking over too
much responsibility for the activity, and the extent to which she is
able to interact with the patient on a personal level. As the
patients' self-care abilities and level of independence varies, so the
way in which the nurse achieves this goal differs. By grouping
patients according to their need for nursing assistance and

identifying the most appropriate helping methods, the prescribed nursing requirements for a range of patients can be compared to the actual nurse activity and patient outcomes, and the extent to which the actual activity meets the prescribed goals can, therefore, be determined. When the observed activity meets the prescribed goal, the interaction is therapeutic and provides optimal care; if the observed activity fails, however, to meet the prescribed goal, it is less therapeutic and of poorer quality.

It was on such a premise that the framework with which to classify and code the quality of nurse activity and patient outcomes was based. The framework had as its theoretical background the concepts that had been developed in the TNF indicator and, earlier, in the theoretical framework for geriatric nursing. The framework began by describing the three main nursing systems used to identify patients' needs for assistance; the prescribed nursing care goals were then identified for each of the patients being studied in Brown and White Wards, and, finally, a coding system was developed that graded patient involvement, nursing activity and patient outcomes according to their level of therapeutic content.

### Nursing systems

The identification of nursing systems in the evaluation of quality of care relates to the overall theoretical framework for nursing developed in the study. Rather than define patients' needs according to medical model characteristics, for example, whether patients are assessment, rehabilitation or continuing care, a nursing framework was used. This helped to focus attention on nursing's caring contribution rather than reflecting medical observations, which could bias the nurse's assessment of the patient's need for nursing assistance.

According to Orem (1980), nursing systems clarify the scope of the nursing responsibility in health-care systems by identifying both the general and specific roles of the nurses and patients. They also make clear the kind of actions to be performed and the performance pattern of nurses' and patients' actions in regulating patients' self-care capabilities. The three nursing systems identified are based on the principle that nurses, patients, or both nurses and patients, can act to meet patients' self-care requirements and, thus, fulfil the goal of achieving optimal self-care. Patients are grouped into one of three nursing systems, depending on their self-care abilities and potential and their need for certain types of nursing assistance. The systems are wholly compensatory, partly compensatory and supportive–educative.

Patients in the wholly compensatory nursing system are those who are unable to control their position and movement, are unresponsive to most stimuli and are unable to monitor the environment or convey information to others because of loss of motor ability. The consequences for such patients are confinement to one location within the ward, the need for protection from environmental hazards and that all or the majority of decisions regarding self-care are made for them. The most appropriate type of nursing action for this group would be acting and doing for the patient. The nurse would aim to meet patients's self-care needs and compensate for their inability to engage in self-care by supporting and protecting them and providing a non-hazardous or therapeutic environment. Patients would require either continuous or frequent contact and sensitive treatment because of their total dependence on nursing staff.

Patients in the partly compensatory nursing system are able to perform self-care activities but still require assistance. Such patients are aware of themselves and their own environment and are able to communicate with others, yet are usually unable to move about without support or assistance. They may be mentally competent and capable of making decisions about their own self-care, although help may be required to carry out such actions. The most appropriate methods of nursing assistance for such patients would be the maintenance of a therapeutic environment, acting and doing certain tasks for the patient, providing psychological support, guidance and direction in order to build up the patient's self-confidence and, finally, teaching the patient how to cope with an altered set of capabilities. The nurse's interaction with patients in this category should include more discussion about preferred methods of self-care, more diversional activities and co-ordination of care with physio- and occupational therapists. It would also entail a realistic assessment of future functional capacities and shared planning with the patient.

The final nursing system relates to those patients who are able to accomplish self-care but who require supervision and guidance from staff. The most appropriate types of nursing action in this system are the provision and maintenance of a therapeutic

**Table 28**  Nursing systems in geriatric care (after Orem, 1980)

| | Wholly compensatory nursing system | Partly compensatory nursing system | Supportive–educative nursing system |
|---|---|---|---|
| Character-istics of patients | Patients are unable to control position movement in space Unresponsive to stimuli Unable to monitor the environment and convey information to others because of loss of motor ability | Patients are aware of themselves and immediate environment and are able to communicate with others Unable to move about/perform manipulative movements because of restrictions May be mentally competent, capable of making accurate observations May be involved in making judgments and decisions about self-care | Patients are conscious but are unable to focus attention on themselves or others for the purpose of self-care Require guidance and support to make decisions Can ambulate and perform some measures of self-care with certain guidance and supervision |
| Nursing role | Acts in place of and for the patient Provides a therapeutic environment | Maintains a developmental environment Acts in place of and for the patients Provides psychological support Gives guidance and direction Teaches Promotes a normal life-style | Provides and maintains a therapeutic environment Guides and directs Provides support – psychologically, physically and emotionally |
| Patient role | As recipient of care aimed to meet the self-care needs of the patient Actions of nurse compensate for patient's own limitations | Performs some self-care measures Is involved in planning and organising of self-care Accepts care and assistance from nurses | Needs to be willing to be guided and taught how to perform activities |

*(continues overleaf)*

**Table 28**  *continued*

|  | Wholly compensatory nursing system | Partly compensatory nursing system | Supportive-educative nursing system |
|---|---|---|---|
| Nursing action | Speaks to patients using conversational tone<br>Handles patients gently<br>Maintains continuous and frequent contact<br>Maintains environmental conditions that protect and support normal functioning | Discussion with patient about preferred methods of self-care<br>Involves patient in diversional activities<br>Engages in realistic assessment of future function and shared planning with patient | Providing some sort of reality orientation<br>Trying not to let patients retreat into own world<br>Diversional therapy<br>Social interaction |

environment, guiding, directing and supporting the patient. This may take the form of providing some sort of reality orientation or retaining programme for confused patients or patients suffering from functional and mobility limitations. It also includes diversional therapy and social interaction. Table 28 summarises the main features of each nursing system, identifying the nurse's and patient's role in the system as well as outlining the most appropriate type of nursing action to ensure optimal self-care.

The outlines were used to classify patients in Brown and White Ward according to their self-care requirements and nursing needs. This meant that the rehabilitation and continuing care labels could be discarded and that patients could be compared in terms of their need for nursing assistance. Of the eight patients chosen for the study in Brown Ward, three were in the wholly compensatory category, two in the partly compensatory category and three in the supportive–educative group. Three patients in both White and Red Wards were in the wholly compensatory category, four patients in the partly compensatory category and one in the supportive–educative nursing system (see appendix VIIIc Kitson 1984 for detailed information).

The classification of patients into one of three nursing systems, which outlined the role and function of both the nurse and the patient, helped the researcher to determine the prescribed care goals for each patient. Nursing information on the ward in the form of nursing plans and Kardexes was also used to determine the prescribed care goals of each of the patients being observed.

## Nursing care prescriptions

The ability of the nurse to provide care at a level that would meet patients' individual requirements depended on her knowledge of the abilities and limitations of the patient and her ability to identify and provide the most appropriate type of nursing assistance. Nursing records were consulted to determine how much information the nursing staff had about the capabilities of each patient in order to prescribe nursing care goals. The information on patients in Brown Ward (low scoring TNF ward) was compared to the type of information available to nursing staff on White Ward (high scoring TNF ward).

*Wholly compensatory patients.* Within this category, patients in both Brown and White Wards were heavily dependent on nursing staff. Patients were all in their late 80s, suffered from multiple pathological conditions and were immobile. The majority were confused. Information related to the nursing care of the patients in Brown Ward was found in the nursing Kardex and was made up of short comments on the personal hygiene, pressure area care, toilet needs, nutritional, fluid and mobilisation needs of patients. The information in the majority of areas was found to be insufficient to determine the self-care potential of patients and was also found to be inaccurate and out of date. It did not provide personal details either about patients' likes or dislikes or about their self-care limitations. For example, the nutritional needs of each patient were described as a 'normal soft diet', one patient needing to be fed, the others managing with help. Ward observation showed that none of the patients could feed independently and that two of the patients could have become more independent had they been provided with the proper utensils.

In White Ward, although a similar nursing Kardex system was used, much more detailed information was found in relation to patients' personal preferences, and comments were made about how nurses should aim to assist patients in certain self-care activities. An example of the difference between the information available for John A in Brown Ward and Florence B in White ward

**Table 29**  Wholly compensatory patients – nursing care plans

|  | Brown Ward<br>John A | White Ward<br>Florence B |
|---|---|---|
| Age | 92 | 84 |
| Length of hospitalisation | 3 years | 3 years |
| Diagnosis | Mild parkinsonism<br>Confusional state | Hemiplegia<br>Aphasia |
| Personal hygiene | Dependent, needs help to wash | Dependent on staff; weekly bath, encourage to assist; likes hair set |
| Dressing/undressing | – | Dependent on staff (uses hospital clothes washed by unit); apply pad and bandage to R heel at night |
| Toilet needs | Toilet 3-hourly; uses urinal with help; needs help to toilet | Toiletted 2-hourly during day, 4-hourly at night; incontinent of urine at times |
| Nutrition | Normal soft diet | Normal diet; needs food cut up; uses melamine plate with antislip mat; normal cutlery; encourage fluids |
| Mobility | Chairfast; passive exercises may be carried out | Left leg very contracted; care when lifting – unable to stand/walk; needs two to transfer from bed to chair |
| Comments | – | Concentration poor; encourage to talk, loves flowers, likes chair to face window so that she can look out into the street |

is given in table 29. Additional information about John A, which would have been important in organising and planning nurisng care but which was not given in the Kardex, was that he had cataracts in both eyes, which severely limited his field of vision. However, nothing was said about his poor eyesight in relation to his ability to feed himself or to the type of nursing assistance he would require to ensure that he would not be deprived of information because of his visual handicap.

This trend of poor nursing information was carried through each of the other care plans for wholly compensatory patients in Brown Ward. In contrast, the care plans for patients in White Ward with similar disabilities to those in Brown Ward appeared to be much more illuminating in terms of their self-care abilities, limitations, likes and dislikes. Information was not readily available to nurses on Brown Ward. Whereas additional information was available to nurses in the medical case notes, there was very little detail about either the personal likes and dislikes of patients or the ways in which nursing staff could increase patients' self-care potential. In White Ward, although the information on patients' abilities was still limited, the orientation of the care plans was much more patient-centred, detailing particular requirements of patients.

*Partly compensatory patients.* A similar pattern was detected in the type of information available to nursing staff for partly compensatory patients in Brown and White Wards. Patients in this category displayed a range of mobility and functional abilities that required careful documentation if they were to be used and developed by nursing staff. The care plans of the two patients in Brown Ward in this category were no better than the comments that had been noted for patients in the wholly compensatory category. Scant personal detail was provided with which the nurse could determine a patient's self-care potential and nursing requirements. For example, Jack M, who had suffered for several years from rheumatoid arthritis, had been admitted to hospital for investigation of increased immobility and incontinence. The nursing care plan did not comment on Jack's mobility limitations, neither did it indicate that one of the main reasons for his admission to hospital was to investigate his problem of incontinence. Although both medical and paramedical notes gave details of Jack's mobility and functional ability limitations, this information was not conveyed to the nursing staff in the nursing care plan.

Four patients in White Ward were classified in the partly compensatory nursing system. Detailed information was provided about each patient's dressing and washing abilities, and certain food preferences were noted. Information on mobility and elimination needs was also provided in patients' nursing care plans. For example, Margaret N's toilet needs were specifically documented, highlighting the fact that she 'required to be toiletted because she was not always aware of a full bladder'. Patient's likes and dislikes were also noted: Betty K was particularly fond of reading and having visitors, whereas Margaret N, who was rather a reserved individual, enjoyed an occasional chat.

Personal details of patients in Brown Ward were absent in the nursing care plans and were best found in the medical and paramedical notes. Nursing action tended to be limited to acting and doing for patients, with little consideration of their self-care abilities or potential. In contrast, the information on patients in White Ward was more detailed and personal, identifying nursing assistance in terms of helping, supervision, acting for and providing a therapeutic environment.

*Supportive–educative patients.* Three of the eight patients being observed in Brown Ward and one in White Ward belonged to this category. The relative imbalance in this category reflected the overall numbers in the two wards, Brown Ward having a larger number of patients who were more independent in self-care needs. All the patients in this category required guidance, support and teaching from nursing staff in order to improve their self-care potentials.

Two of the patients in Brown Ward, Sam M and Joseph D, had undergone treatment from physio- and occupational therapists, which should have been reinforced and practised in the ward setting. The other two patients – both elderly ladies in their late 80s, who suffered from mild intermittent attacks of confusion – were supported by the ward staff through the provision of a routine that met their self-care needs. The nurse's therapeutic function for such patients, however, should have been the provision of a therapeutic environment, encouraging the patients to remain as independent as possible while knowing how best to deal with periods of confusion.

For Sam M and Joseph D, the aim of hospitalisation was to develop mobility and functional ability to a level that would enable them to return to the community. Their nursing care plans, however, displayed a lack of detailed comment that would have enabled members of the nursing team to know how to meet the self-care needs of either patient. No information was available on Sam M's care plan concerning his level of mobility or functional ability, for example, whether he could use a knife and fork or whether he required his food to be cut up. Similarly, Joseph D's care plan lacked any measure of detail or indication of his self-care capacity. Joseph, a man in his 80s, had been admitted as an emergency case, suffering from a chest infection, dehydration, confusion, immobility and incontinence. After the initial acute stage, the medical goal for Joseph was to rehabilitate him and get him back home, which meant sorting out his immobility and continence problems. However, the nursing care plan neither made staff aware of the medical goal nor elucidated the patient's potential for achieving such a goal. Joseph's toilet needs were described as 'use of urinal, commode chair to toilet' whereas mobilisation needs consisted of 'gets up to sit in chair, can stand only'. A description of the nurse's contribution towards encouraging and re-educating Joseph in the performance of these self-care measures was absent.

The information available to staff in Brown Ward for patients in the supportive–educative category was general and unspecific. It did not provide staff with an indication of patients' self-care potential, nor did it provide them with directives as to how to support and teach patients. This problem was repeated for each category of patient in Brown Ward. Very little detailed information was given about any patient, and nursing staff tended to provide the same sort of care to all patients, irrespective of the nursing system to which they belonged. For example, the prescription for the treatment of pressure areas was the same for each patient regardless of their level of continence, mobility, hydration, nutritional state and level of mental awareness. More information about patients' self-care abilities was found in medical and paramedical notes than in the nursing records in Brown Ward, and this information was used by the researcher to determine the actual self-care potential of patients and to ensure that they had been placed in the correct nursing system.

Nursing staff in White Ward, on the other hand, received more information about patients' self-care abilities, which were described in terms of the types of aid and the nursing support they required. The likes and dislikes were documented, along with particular interests and hobbies. Medical and paramedical notes provided little additional information about patients, and the care plans were found to reflect accurately patients' self-care abilities.

A consideration of patients' nursing care plans identified particular requirements of those patients being observed on the ward and enabled the researcher to form an opinion as to the most appropriate type of prescribed care required to meet the goal of optimal self-care. The fact that patient and nurse roles were defined in the nursing systems meant that a baseline could be set for measuring the quality of nurse actions and patient outcomes in the ward setting. The next step in the methodology was to develop a scale that would grade self-care activities into therapeutic or less therapeutic action, depending on whether the sequence of events led to the prescribed outcome, i.e. the provision of optimal self-care and independence, or whether it resulted in an underutilisation of the patient's self-care abilities and a loss of independence and dignity.

### Grading self-care activities – the TNF matrix

The goal of care was seen to be the maintenance of the patient at the optimal level of self-care. Actions, therefore, that overlooked the patient's capabilities or did not encourage him to use certain self-care skills were seen as non-therapeutic. Also, nursing activity that denied the patient the opportunity of making decisions about his self-care was seen as non-therapeutic, as were actions that made him more dependent. Lack of encouragement, lack of knowledge of patients' conditions and lack of stimulation and teaching of certain patients was seen as non-therapeutic, as was the failure to provide patients with privacy or to maintain their dignity during the performance of certain procedures.

An attempt was made to construct a scaling system that would grade the level of therapeutic content of nursing action and patient outcomes for each of the three nursing systems. The resulting TNF matrix (see appendix VII) divided each self-care activity into three phases – initiation, process and outcome. The initiation phase concentrated on the initiation of the action. This could have been patient-initiated, initiated with nursing assistance or initiated directly by the nurse. If the nurse responded to the patient's requests for assistance or anticipated his need for assistance, the initiation was seen as therapeutic and given a numerical rating of 4 points. If the nurse initiated the interaction without the prior knowledge or consent of the patient, the activity was seen as non-therapeutic and was awarded 1 point. If the patient initiated the request for assistance and the nurse responded promptly in a manner that maintained the patient's optimal level of independence, her action was seen as positive facilitation and therapeutic. Conversely, when an activity had been poorly initiated and the nurse had not attempted to obtain the patient's co-operation, the facilitation was seen as poor.

Consideration of a patient's elimination needs serves as an example of how the initiation phase of an activity was observed and graded for therapeutic content. Martha O was a fairly independent patient in the supportive–educative category. From her mobility and functional ability assessment, she would have been expected to meet her elimination needs independently (awarded 4 points). If she received assistance from the nurse that was helpful but not particularly necessary, the initiation phase would be awarded 3 points because the nurse had not taken full account of the patient's self-care capabilities and potential. A score of 2 on the TNF matrix was given when the nurse initiated the activity with little explanation to and co-operation from the patient, and a score of 1 point was reserved for those interactions initiated by the nurse without the co-operation of the patient. An example of this would have been toiletting an ambulant patient like Martha by wheeling her to the toilet as part of the routine toilet round rather than as a response to a request from the patient.

The second stage of the TNF scaling matrix was termed the process stage. It involved making a judgment on the effectiveness of the performance of the self-care action and, if she was directly involved, on whether or not the nurse was using her knowledge and skills to help to develop or maintain the patient's optimal level of self-care. If the nurse was not directly involved in the self-care activity, e.g. Martha O going to the toilet independently, the process was evaluated in relation to the ease with which the patient could carry out the task within the environment.

Three areas of patient activity were considered in the process stage: the level at which the patient was able to utilise functional abilities; mobility potential and limitations; and whether aids and appliances were provided that would safeguard or improve the patient's level of independence. Each patient's mobility and functional ability levels had to be known before an assessment could be made as to whether or not the nurse had properly taken account of these abilities and had performed or facilitated the task accordingly. For example, a patient in the partly compensatory category engaged in the process of feeding might have had functional limitations relating to his mobility limitations, such as a paralysed right arm, and limited eyesight, which made independence in feeding more difficult. This patient, however, might be independent in feeding if provided with the correct appliances, such as a non-slip mat for his plate or a plate with detachable sides, as an aid to one-handed feeding. He might also need his food cut up into manageable portions before he could be left to eat his meal unaided. The nurse's therapeutic function in this situation would be to ensure that the patient is able to achieve an optimal level of independence with the help of a variety of aids and feeding gadgets. In this example, the process state would obtain a maximum of 4 points when the patient is able to feed independently with the aid of appropriate feeding utensils. When the nurse fails to utilise the patient's optimal mobility and functional abilities and does not attempt to provide environmental aids, the process score would range from 3 points to 1 point, depending on how poorly the activity was performed.

The final section of the matrix considered the outcome of the activity. This was linked directly to the goal content, which for every patient was the achievement of optimal self-care and independence. A successful outcome for a patient in the supportive–educative system could have been meeting his elimination needs by deciding to go to the toilet, walking from the day-room to the toilet, using the toilet unaided and returning to the day-room. For a wholly compensatory patient a therapeutic outcome could have been when the nurse, detecting a restlessness about the patient, realised that it might have been due to bladder fullness, so brought the patient to the toilet. Through anticipating and acting for the patient, the nurse achieves the goal of continence for her patient. Outcomes of limited or minimal success, or which were unsuccessful, were assessed by the amount of independence each patient was given and the role the nurse had adopted in the interaction. If the nurse had not used the most appropriate set of helping skills, the outcome for the patient was likely to be less therapeutic.

The TNF matrix was used to grade observations that had been written down in long-hand in the observation schedule. Comments on each nursing activity noted at the time had, therefore, to be sufficiently detailed to enable a judgment to be made as to the therapeutic content of the action at all three stages. Breaking each activity into three stages ensured that the quality of each interaction was considered according to the same basic criteria. Thus, for Joseph D (patient 8 on the observation schedule, appendix IV) coding of the quality of his feeding activities took the following factors into consideration: that he had limited eyesight; that he had a certain amount of cogwheel rigidity associated with mild Parkinsonism; that his self-care potential was high given correct positioning; and the provision of certain feeding aids (for example, a feeding cup with a spout instead of a teacup enabled him to be independent in drinking, and positioning him at a table with his meal at a manageable distance ensured independence in feeding). Joseph's experiences, however, were quite different. The observation schedule (appendix IV) note that Joseph was left in bed to eat breakfast and that an ordinary teacup was placed in front of him on a cantilever table at about chest height. Porridge was put out on a plate, and a spoon left on the cantilever table. No attempt was made by nursing staff to check that Joseph could see where the spoon and the porridge were, never mind considering whether or not he could manage to feed himself given his relatively awkward position in relation to the cantilever table. The result was that Joseph made no attempt to feed himself. In the end, two members of staff, at different times, fed him his porridge. He was then left in bed with the teacup precariously held in his unsteady hand, but after a short time this was taken from him. The outcome was that the half-full cup of tea was taken from him and set on the cantilever table out of reach; no attempt was made to offer Joseph a more appropriate drinking vessel.

Relating these observations to the TNF matrix, the initiation of the activity was given one point on the scale as no attempt had been made by the nurse to ascertain what Joseph required to make him as independent as possible in this activity. The process stage was also poor in that the facilities available to the nurse to help the patient achieve optimal independence not made use of – Joseph was left sitting uncomfortably in bed, the cantilever table was at an awkward height, the teacup was an inappropriate drinking vessel. The outcome, predictably, was poor, the activity being non-therapeutic for Joseph. Thus, the coding of Joseph's feeding activity resulted in a series of low scores, indicating poor nursing anticipation and action, resulting in underutilisation of the patient's self-care potential. The numerical coding for this activity was:

| Column | 1 | 2 | 3 | 4 | 5 |
|---|---|---|---|---|---|
| Observation | 0 | 2 | 1 | 1 | 1 |

Columns 1 and 2 relate to the activity code (appendix V), whereas columns 3, 4 and 5 provide information on the quality of the initiation, process and outcome of the activity. An activity such as feeding could have spanned several observation units. In order to ensure that the therapeutic content of each observation was documented, the initiation, process and outcome scores were noted in each unit of observation. Thus, for Joseph, whose breakfast spanned four units of observations (a time period of 16 minutes from when it was served until the breakfast dishes were cleared away), although the initiation phase related to the first unit of observation, the information was carried into each of the following observations until the whole activity terminated:

Quantity and quality score of feeding observations for Joseph D

| Time | Activity quality |
|------|------------------|
| 8.00 | 0 2 1 1 1 |
| 8.06 | 0 2 1 1 1 |
| 8.12 | 0 2 1 1 1 |
| 8.18 | 0 2 1 1 1 |

This meant that when data were analysed according to self-care activity or patient type, both the quantity and quality of interactions would remain intact.

## Nursing staff

Although nursing action was being graded according to its therapeutic content, no attempt was made to identify those members of staff who gave more therapeutic care and those who gave less therapeutic nursing care. The aim was to look at and evaluate nursing action on the ward as a whole, the total level of therapeutic care reflecting the orientation of the ward sister and her level of therapeutic awareness rather than the individual orientation of nursing staff. Thus, in Brown Ward, where the ward sister had a low TNF score, one would expect lower levels of therapeutic activity from staff, whereas in White Ward, where the ward sister had a high TNF score, one would expect to find significantly higher levels of therapeutic activity.

It was felt, however, that individual staff members should to have the opportunity to comment on their work and, particularly, on what they thought of the system of assessing, planning and implementing care on the ward. Consequently each member of staff on Brown and White Ward was interviewed by the researcher at the end of the observation exercise (see appendix IXe in Kitson,

1984). Generally, staff were very responsive and spoke readily of their feelings about work and its organisation. The information enabled the researcher to compare staff views with those of the ward sisters to see if the orientations of the ward sister did have an effect on the individual experiences and had perceptions of nursing staff.

Ward sisters were also interviewed at this time, although much of the same sort of information had been collected using the TNF indicator. The interview, however, served as an opportunity for the ward sister to elaborate on any aspect of care on the ward. A total of 20 staff was interviewed in Brown Ward – comprising the ward sister, four SRNs, one SEN, eight student nurses and six nursing auxiliaries. In White Ward, 16 day-duty staff were interviewed – the ward sister, three SRNs, two SENs, three student nurses and seven nursing auxiliaries.

## FINDINGS – COMPARISON OF BROWN AND WHITE WARDS

Both wards had a ward profile score (WPS) of 60.1, which indicated moderate facilities; ancillary services were provided by the main hospital departments, whereas the geriatric unit had its own physiotherapy, occupational therapy department and personalised laundry system. The consultant geriatrician visited the unit once per week, his deputies visiting more frequently or on requests from the sister. From the medical perspectivie, Brown Ward was designated an assessment and rehabilitation ward, although, in reality, a significant proportion of its patients, particularly its male patients; were continuing care. White Ward was designated as continuing care, although, when there were no beds available in Brown Ward, so-called assessment and rehabilitation patients were admitted. Thus, despite the different medical designation, the general mobility and functional ability levels of patients in Brown and White Ward were similar (see appendix VIIIc in Kitson, 1984). The main difference was that Brown Ward was a mixed male and female ward and White Ward was a female ward.

## Staff – ward sister (see appendix III)

Sister 'Brown' in Brown Ward, who had a TNF score of 83, tended to view her work as the provision of basic nursing care, supplemented by a kind and sympathetic approach to patients' individual problems. Although she perceived herself as someone who was aware of the social and emotional aspects of patient care, she did not have an organised system for collecting such information from patients. Patients' self-care needs were not documented in any great detail, and nursing staff were not provided with individual care plans. The communication of information on the ward began with the morning report given by night staff to sister and trained staff, during which time nursing auxiliaries commenced serving breakfast. Staff were not told what to do for patients but were expected to organise themselves and get on with the work. Rarely were they required to report back to sister on patients' conditions.

Trained nurses did not require specialist training in caring for the elderly, according to Sister Brown, and the nurse's role in the rehabilitation of patients related to knowing how to walk patients. Sister Brown tended to see rehabilitation as the responsibility of paramedical workers, something that nursing staff should know about but which did not really involve them. She felt that the multidisciplinary ward round was not very useful, commenting that the consultant would rather have nurses 'out on the ward with the patients in case they fell.'

Sister Brown did not appear to have distinguished between her nursing role and the medical goal for patients. The overall aim for patients on her ward appeared to be rehabilitation and possible discharge, together with care of the inevitable 'failures', the continuing care patients. Very little detailed information was available to nursing staff, who did not appear to be encouraged to find out about patients' conditions. Work was organised according to a well-established routine, sister feeling confident that patients' needs were being met and that she was fulfilling her role as an assistant to the medical goal of rehabilitation and discharge.

Sister 'White' in White Ward had a TNF score of 123. She had become interested in geriatric nursing through her experiences as a ward sister in a general medical ward, where she noticed that after the first week or so of treatment nothing constructive seemed to be done for elderly patients. She chose to go into geriatric nursing as an attempt to practise some positive sort of nursing care.

She believed that the most important part of nursing care was to make patients feel happy and to maintain their dignity. Having to lower her standards of care constantly and not being able to maintain care goals, which in themselves were relatively simple but labour intensive, were sources of great frustration to her. She saw the nurse's role as including a range of skills, stating that a good nurse had to have the skill of a physiotherapist, occupational therapist, social worker and doctor – all in one person! The provision of personal care, observing, documenting and analysing patients' needs were seen as major priorities. Sister also saw her role as an educator and encourager, commenting that her job was to make her staff nurses good enough to maker her redundant!

The attitudes of Sister White were reflected in the way she organised and prescribed work on the ward. Patient assessments were more detailed; staff were encouraged to find out as much as they could about patients, and all members of the nursing team were included in the morning report. This report was given after the night report; trained staff were allocated a group of patients and, with their teams, were responsible for the total care of those patients. Although the sister appeared to have been successful in implementing a more patient-centred approach to care, she did comment on her feelings of disillusionment at times and isolation from colleagues. She felt that none of the sisters on the other geriatric wards shared the same views about patient care and that nursing management was not behind her efforts because she was constantly agitating for improved working conditions and better staffing levels.

*SRNs*
Four SRNs worked on Brown Ward and, from the interviews, two separate orientations were detected in their comments about their work. Two SRNs, both of whom had worked on the ward for over 10 years, felt satisfied with the way work was organised. Geriatric nursing was seen as a vocation, and nurses were supposed to know intuitively what to do for patients. The biggest problem was lack of staff, with the result that staff were unable to spend time chatting with patient or getting them to do things for themselves. One staff nurse explained how the shortage of staff affected her relationship with patients by citing Jack M's case. She said:

'I'm always at him to do things for himself, like button his shirt, because before he came in here he was able to do this himself.'

She concluded, however, by saying that she did not have the time to allow patients like Jack to do things for himself:

'The work is so routinised, it'll never be any different; we're always watching the clock.'

Thus, whereas the SRNs were aware of the need to encourage patients to do things for themselves, they did not appear to see this as a realistic nursing goal, given the staff constraints.

The other two SRNs in Brown Ward held quite different opinions on their role and the organisation of care on the ward. They worked part-time and had been on Brown Ward for less than 2 years. Both commented on their feelings of frustration on the ward as they were rarely given responsibility for patient care or allowed to make decisions and considered that they were used as 'just an extra pair of hands'. They felt that the patient information system was inadequate and nurses, consequently, had to provide care without either a knowledge of paramedical and medical treatment regimens or a nursing assessment of patients' mobility and functional abilities. Both felt that patients were dealt with in a batch manner. One SRN said that she would like to be able to follow through patients' problems and be given more initiative to listen to, counsel and help patients. They felt that the only way the situation could be improved was to provide staff with more individualised patient information.

Three SRNs, one of whom was full-time, worked in White Ward. All were in their late 30s, married and had worked betwen 1 and 3 years in White Ward. None was dissatisfied with the way work was organised on the ward, and they all felt that the sister was very fair and helped to educate all staff on the ward. They were satisfied with the way their skills were being used, one staff nurse commenting that she felt it was necessary that she was out on the ward to teach and supervise student nurses and auxiliary staff. However, none of the staff nurses reflected the breadth of vision of their nursing role in the care of the elderly that had been detected in sister. Although they were happy with the way work was organised, they were unable to articulate in detail the range of nursing activities in which they should be involved.

## SENs

One SEN worked in Brown Ward and two in White Ward. All were part-time, married and had been working on the ward for less than 1 year. The SEN in Brown ward saw her role as the provision of basic nursing care. She did not see it as encompassing the patients' social and emotional needs as she felt elderly people were generally 'too confused' to have emotional needs, whereas nurses were 'too busy' to meet patients' social needs. She considered nursing care to be organised satisfactorily on the ward, given the staff shortages. Although she had little responsibility in the decision-making process for patients, she seemed to be quite happy with this arrangement. She did not really know what patients did at physiotherapy and occupational therapy and did not feel that this was an area of interest to her.

In contrast to the SEN in Brown Ward, one of the SENs in White Ward held a set of totally different perspectives about her role and function in geriatric care. She began by identifying the need for nursing staff to recognise patients' individual requirements and to determine what level of assistance the nurse should provide for the patient. She believed that it was only an experienced and knowledgeable nurse who could judge accurately when and how to meet patients' needs. She also mentioned the sensitivity that nurses required in caring for the elderly, to be able to gauge certain situations when, for example, patients need someone to sit down and talk to them.

She felt that geriatric nursing was much more than tender loving care and required a knowledge of how far to push the patient towards independence and self care. It was not just a question of common sense in knowing how to meet the needs of old people; rather it was a specialised task that should be the expertise of a trained geriatric nurse. She also expressed the importance of building up close and meaningful relationships with elderly patients and of knowing how to use group dynamics as a therapeutic tool in stimulating patients in the ward environment. She saw rehabilitation as an integral part of nursing and not as an activity carried out solely by paramedical staff – it was a process of giving the right assistance and encouragement at the right time.

She was satisfied with the way work was organised on the ward and felt that the ward sister was excellent in motivating staff. She felt that the routine of the ward had to be flexible enough to enable nursing staff to do such things as sit down and talk to patients, rather than rushing around doing other tasks. According to this SEN, one of the most satisfying activities in the care of old people was to be able to show patients what they could do for themselves.

## Student nurses

Brown ward had three final-year student nurses and three first-years, whereas White ward had three students on their first ward experience. First-year nurses on both wards tended to describe geriatric nursing as 'hard work' and 'fun at times', but said it was not 'real nursing' – real nursing was giving injections and caring for medical and surgical patients.

The third-year student nurses, who were completing an 8-week period on Brown Ward, were more articulate. The general feeling was that work on Brown Ward was disorganised and confusing. Nurses were not told what to do for patients, team leaders were not delegated responsibility and students felt that trained staff expected them to know what to do. One student described how she had to pick up information about patients' capabilities in bits and pieces rather than be told about them. She gave the example of Sam M, saying that it was only by accident that she discovered he was to be rehabilitated for eventual discharge home. After this, she began to encourage him to do more things for himself. Another student recounted similar frustrations in not knowing what patients could do for themselves. For example, she said she had been wheeling Minnie W to the toilet each morning until she discovered Minnie could walk!

## Nursing auxiliaries

The six nursing auxiliaries in Brown Ward ranged in age and experience from one 18-year-old who had just started working in the ward to an auxiliary in her 50s who had worked there for several years. As a group, the auxiliaries were least forthcoming in their comments and opinions about work. Whereas they said they really liked working with the elderly, some felt dissatisfied at the way they were treated. They were unhappy about not being included in the nursing report sessions, with the result that they knew very little about patients' general nursing needs. They also felt that they had been ill-prepared for their work. Such situations tended to build up feelings of resentment and frustration, and these were detected in some of the nursing auxiliaries' comments.

The majority of nursing auxiliary staff in White Ward were in their 40s and had worked on the ward between 6 months and 2 years. They all commented on how much they enjoyed the contact with patients and being able to do things for them. They found that the sister was very helpful and supportive, mentioning how she had taught them such procedures as 'lifting patients without hurting your back', 'how to feed patients' and 'how to move them in chairs'. They were generally content with their work role and felt they had been given adequate training by the sister. They also thought that they were provided with sufficient information on patients' conditions to be able to meet their individual needs.

## Comments

There seemed to be two groups of nurses spanning both wards; one group was routine-centred whereas the other was patient-centred. The routine-centred nurses in Brown Ward were content with the way in which care was organised and saw their role in terms of doing for and acting on behalf of patients. This approach reflected Sister Brown's views and was the predominant force on the ward. In White Ward two SRNs and one SEN appeared to have the same routine approach, although it was masked by the prevalent attitudes of Sister White. Whereas these staff said they preferred the patient-centred approach adopted on ward, they also expressed reservations about the realism of such an approach, commenting on how hard Sister White worked for so little return.

Those who did not accept the routine approach to patient care included several nurses in Brown Ward, unhappy and frustrated by the way care was organized, and one SEN in White Ward who shared Sister White's positive and patient-centred approach to care. Although SRNs, students and nursing auxiliary staff were dissatisfied with the way work was organised in Brown Ward, they seemed to be powerless to alter the general approach from routine-dominated care to a preferred patient-centred orientation. Conversely, staff in White Ward who displayed less commitment to the patient-centred approach still carried out their work in a more patient-aware way. Thus, despite the fact that both wards contained staff who favoured both routine- and patient-centred care, the overall care orientation in the ward seemed to depend on the ward sister's approach to patient welfare.

In White Ward all staff, including those nurses who were not fully convinced of its effectiveness in the practice situation, were expected and trained to provide more patient-centred care. The outcome was a more contented group of workers, able to describe quite clearly a range of nursing skills and activities that were part of their nursing care. Staff in Brown Ward either concurred with sister's more limited perspective of nursing, and saw their work in terms of the provision of routine basic care requiring few skills and little training, or else they rejected this approach. Those who rejected Sister Brown's approach found themselves frustrated by the ward routine but powerless to effect any change. This situation, in which a significant number of staff in Brown Ward found themselves, underlined the belief that it was the ward sister's orientation to the care of her patients, rather than the individual perspectives of staff, that determined the overall standard.

### Time spent in self-care and other activities on Brown Ward and White Ward

Patients' activities were divided into three main areas: activities relating to self-care – elimination, feeding, drink, washing, bathing, dressing, undressing, exercising and communicating; time spent with other members of the multidisciplinary team – doctors, physiotherapists, occupational therapists; and time spent by themselves in the day-room, in the ward bays or in bed. The amount of time spent by patients on each activity was determined by adding the number of observations for each action and dividing by the total number of observations per patient. This figure was then converted to a percentage of the total number of observations. Table 30 shows the proportion of time spent in self-care activities, in contact with other professionals and in inactivity for the eight patients in Brown Ward compared with the eight patients in White Ward.

Observation of self-care activity included the whole cycle of events related to the initiation, performance and completion of the action. For example, observation of a patient's feeding activities would commence with the initial contact of the nurse in providing the patient with the meal and would end when the patient had finished or when the utensils were cleared away. Observation of elimination, washing, dressing and undressing activities was similarly based on the initiation, performance and completion or termination of the action. Sometimes a whole sequence would take less than 1 minute; others lasted several minutes.

**Table 30.** Time devoted to self-care and other activities in Brown and White Wards

|  | Brown Ward (%) | White Ward (%) |
|---|---|---|
| **Self-care activities** | | |
| Elimination | 3.3 | 4.6 |
| Feeding | 8.1 | 8.2 |
| Drinking | 2.6 | 2.5 |
| Washing | 1.4 | 1.9 |
| Bathing | 0.3 | 0.3 |
| Dressing | 1.5 | 1.4 |
| Undressing | 1.1 | 1.4 |
| Exercising | 1.7 | 1.8 |
| Communicating | 1.7 | 3.0 |
| *Total* | 21.7 | 25.1 |
| **Contact** | | |
| Doctors | 0.1 | 0.1 |
| Physiotherapists | 2.3 | 2.0 |
| Occupational therapists | 1.1 | 0.3 |
| Others | 1.7 | 0.6 |
| Visitors | 3.1 | 4.1 |
| *Total* | 7.3 | 7.1 |
| **Inactive** | | |
| Day-room | 21.5 | 12.4 |
| Ward bay | 26.3 | 40.6 |
| Bed | 21.1 | 13.8 |
| Other | 3.0 | 1.1 |
| *Total* | 71.9 | 67.9 |

Observation of patients' exercising and communication activities required more detailed definition. Exercise was divided into three categories: first, it could involve the passive exercising of patients' limbs by nursing staff and, second, it could occur when a nurse chose to assist the patient in the performance of another self-care activity in such a way that practice was given in walking or exercising part of the body, e.g. a nurse choosing to walk the patient to the toilet or day-room rather than wheel him in a chair. The final activity coded under exercise was the patient practising mobility skills without nursing assistance or encouragement. Exercise did not include mobility activity carried out by paramedical staff in the physiotherapy unit.

Only verbal communication that was observed taking place outside an interaction between the nurse and the patient was included under the communication heading. Observations were also divided into communication that was nurse-initiated and communication that was patient-initiated, which could relate to either general topics or to specific requests in respect of self-care action.

Just over one-fifth of patients' time was taken up with self-care activities in Brown Ward, compared to one-quarter of patients' time in White Ward. Most time was devoted to feeding activities, with elimination needs being the next most time-consuming activity for both wards. Each of the remaining self-care activities took up between 1 and 2% of patients' time, patients in White Ward communicating slightly more often than those in Brown Ward. The difference between the amount of time spent on self-care activities on either ward was not found to be statistically significant ($\chi^2$ = 0.1034, $p$ >0.05).

Contact with other members of the multidisciplinary team was infrequent for patients on both wards; relatives made up most of the contact, whereas doctors had least contact. Approximately 2% of patients' time in both wards was taken up with physiotherapy contact. Patients in Brown Ward spent proportionally more time in bed than did patients in White Ward, although, again, the difference between the two observations was not statistically significant ($\chi^2$ = 1.1372, $p$ > 0.05).

The amount of time spent on self-care activities, in contact with other personnel and in relative inactivity for patients in wholly compensatory, partly compensatory and supportive–educative nursing systems on the two wards is shown in table 31.

Patients in the wholly compensatory category had least time spent on their self-care needs in both wards, whereas patients in the partly compensatory category devoted almost one-quarter of their time to these activities. Most time, in all three groups, was spent on feeding. Time spent on elimination needs was lowest for wholly compensatory patients in Brown Ward – 2.9% of total time compared to 4.4% in White Ward.

Partly compensatory patients in Brown Ward spent slightly more time on self-care activities than did supportive–educative patients, whereas in White Ward patients in the supportive–educative category took more time. Contact with members of the multidisciplinary team was low for wholly compensatory patients

**Table 31.** Time devoted to self-care and other activities, by nursing system

| | Wholly compensatory patients | | Partly compensatory patients | | Supportive– educative patients | |
|---|---|---|---|---|---|---|
| | Brown | White | Brown | White | Brown | White |
| **Self-care Activities** | | | | | | |
| Elimination | 2.9 | 4.4 | 5.6 | 5.3 | 2.2 | 2.5 |
| Feeding | 7.9 | 8.8 | 7.3 | 7.8 | 8.8 | 8.0 |
| Drinking | 2.5 | 2.3 | 2.6 | 2.9 | 2.8 | 2.9 |
| Washing | 2.1 | 2.2 | 1.5 | 1.5 | 1.0 | 2.5 |
| Bathing | 0.1 | 0.2 | 0.1 | 0.5 | 0.6 | 0.2 |
| Dressing | 1.1 | 0.8 | 1.6 | 1.2 | 1.8 | 3.8 |
| Undressing | 1.1 | 1.3 | 1.1 | 1.2 | 1.1 | 2.3 |
| Exercising | 0.0 | 0.7 | 2.2 | 2.1 | 3.0 | 4.3 |
| Communicating | 1.4 | 2.2 | 2.8 | 3.3 | 1.3 | 3.0 |
| *Total* | 19.1 | 22.1 | 24.8 | 25.8 | 22.6 | 29.5 |
| **Contact** | | | | | | |
| Doctors | 0.0 | 0.1 | 0.3 | 0.0 | 0.1 | 0.1 |
| Physiotherapists | 0.0 | 1.3 | 2.4 | 1.9 | 4.3 | 5.0 |
| Occupational Therapists | 0.0 | 0.0 | 4.4 | 0.4 | 0.2 | 0.0 |
| Others | 0.2 | 0.1 | 1.3 | 0.9 | 0.5 | 0.2 |
| Visitors | 3.8 | 2.8 | 2.3 | 5.7 | 2.9 | 1.5 |
| *Total* | 4.0 | 4.3 | 10.7 | 8.9 | 8.0 | 6.8 |
| **Inactive** | | | | | | |
| Day-room | 18.5 | 32.7 | 24.2 | 1.8 | 26.2 | 0.0 |
| Ward Bay | 25.5 | 19.4 | 24.0 | 54.1 | 28.7 | 48.9 |
| Bed | 32.1 | 19.8 | 16.1 | 9.3 | 14.5 | 14.7 |
| *Total* | 76.1 | 71.9 | 64.6 | 65.2 | 69.4 | 63.6 |

(in the region of 4%), increasing to 10.7% and 8.9% for partly compensatory patients and 8% and 6.8% for supportive – educative patients on Brown and White Ward.

No significant difference could be found between the amount of time that patients spent in self-care activities on Brown and White Ward. It would appear that there is a general pattern of activities carried out in geriatric wards in which between one-fifth and one-quarter of patients' time is taken up with self-care activities, one-tenth in contact with other members of the multidisciplinary team and the remainder either sitting in the day-room or ward bay or in bed. This time could be spent either inactive or involved in activities such as talking, reading, watching TV, knitting or smoking.

**Table 32** Therapeutic content of self-care activity in Brown and White Wards

| | | Brown Ward | | White Ward | |
|---|---|---|---|---|---|
| | | % score | Weighted score | % score | Weighted score |
| Elimination | 4 | 14.3 | 57.2 | 6.8 | 27.2 |
| | 3 | 13.9 | 41.7 | 55.8 | 167.4 |
| | 2 | 31.4 | 62.8 | 33.8 | 67.6 |
| | 1 | 40.3 | 40.3 | 3.6 | 3.6 |
| Feeding | 4 | 18.4 | 73.6 | 47.1 | 188.4 |
| | 3 | 21.7 | 65.1 | 37.1 | 111.3 |
| | 2 | 25.6 | 31.2 | 10.5 | 21.0 |
| | 1 | 34.3 | 34.3 | 5.2 | 5.2 |
| Washing | 4 | 2.9 | 11.6 | 29.9 | 119.6 |
| | 3 | 6.7 | 20.1 | 22.8 | 68.4 |
| | 2 | 34.6 | 69.2 | 19.7 | 39.4 |
| | 1 | 55.7 | 255.7 | 27.5 | 227.5 |
| Dressing | 4 | 5.8 | 23.2 | 39.8 | 159.2 |
| | 3 | 24.3 | 72.9 | 15.1 | 45.3 |
| | 2 | 24.3 | 48.6 | 40.9 | 81.8 |
| | 1 | 45.6 | 45.6 | 4.3 | 4.3 |
| Undressing | 4 | 2.7 | 10.8 | 26.1 | 104.4 |
| | 3 | 37.3 | 111.9 | 28.3 | 84.9 |
| | 2 | 30.7 | 61.4 | 33.7 | 67.4 |
| | 1 | 29.3 | 29.3 | 11.9 | 11.9 |
| Exercising | 4 | 11.4 | 45.6 | 17.8 | 71.2 |
| | 3 | 82.5 | 247.5 | 68.6 | 205.8 |
| | 2 | 2.6 | 5.2 | 12.7 | 25.4 |
| | 1 | 3.5 | 3.5 | 0.8 | 0.8 |
| Communication | | | | | |
| Patient-initiated | 2 | 57.3 | 114.6 | 12.9 | 25.8 |
| | 1 | 13.7 | 13.7 | 13.4 | 13.4 |
| Nurse-initiated | 2 | 22.2 | 44.4 | 49.8 | 99.6 |
| | 1 | 6.8 | 6.8 | 23.9 | 23.9 |

N.B. Bathing activities were excluded as they could not be graded according to therapeutic content.

## Therapeutic content of patients' self-care activities in Brown and White Wards

When the quality of self-care activities was contrasted, a number of interesting variations occurred between the two wards. Table 32 shows the quality scores for each self-care activity achieved by each ward, expressed in terms of the percentage of observations of that activity. The degree of therapeutic content of a self-care

**Table 33** Therapeutic content of self-care activities – summary scores

| Activity | Brown Ward | White Ward | $\chi^2$ | $p$ |
|---|---|---|---|---|
| Elimination | 202 | 266 | 8.48 | 0.004 |
| Feeding | 204 | 326 | 27.62 | 0.000 |
| Washing | 157 | 255 | 22.53 | 0.000 |
| Dressing | 190 | 291 | 20.79 | 0.000 |
| Undressing | 213 | 269 | 6.57 | 0.010 |
| Exercising | 302 | 303 | 1.3265 | 0.248 |
| Communication | | | | |
| Patient | 128 | 39 | 46.37 | 0.000 |
| Nurse | 51 | 123 | 28.971 | 0.000 |

activity was judged using the TNF matrix (see appendix VII) and the patients' prescribed care plans. The self-care activity could either have been performed by the patient independently, with support from the nurse or by the nurse with assistance from the patient. Each activity had been given three scores, relating to the initiation, process and outcome stages. The scores, therefore, could range from 0,0,1 to 4,4,4. These were converted to a single score ranging from optimally therapeutic activity (4 points) to non-therapeutic activity (1 point) as follows:

$$\text{Therapeutic} \quad 4 = 3,3,4{-}4,4,4$$
$$3 = 2,2,3{-}3,3,3$$
$$2 = 1,1,2{-}2,2,2$$
$$\text{Non-therapeutic} \quad 1 = 0,0,1{-}1,1,1$$

The number of observations that were awarded 4, 3, 2 or 1 points on the TNF matrix was then computed to give the frequency of therapeutic function on Brown and White Ward (table 32). Patients' therapeutic levels were also related to their nursing system (see appendixes VIII and IX).

Self-care activities for patients in White Ward were found to be performed in a more therapeutic way. The proportion of activities awarded a top score of 4 points was greater in White Ward for feeding, washing, dressing, undressing, exercising, and nurse-initiated communication. Conversely, the proportion of non-therapeutic activities observed in White Ward was much less than that in Brown Ward. In order to clarify the results and to identify the overall level of therapeutic content of each of the activities, a weighting scale was introduced. Thus, activities had been classed as most therapeutic were multiplied by 4, those in the next category by 3, in the next by 2 and those in the non-therapeutic category by 1 (see column 2, table 32). The result was that a total score for the therapeutic content of the self-care activities performed on each ward could be determined (table 33).

This method was also used to compare the overall level of therapeutic activity in relation to the wholly compensatory, partly compensatory and supportive-educative categories (table 34).

There was a significant difference between Brown and White Ward in the quality of elimination, feeding, washing, dressing and

**Table 34** Scores for therapeutic content of self-care activities, by nursing systems

| Activity | | Brown Ward | White Ward | $\chi^2$ | $p$ |
|---|---|---|---|---|---|
| Elimination | WC | 165 | 247 | 15.92 | 0.000 |
| | PC | 226 | 261 | 2.37 | 0.120 |
| | SE | 209 | 400 | 59.28 | 0.000 |
| Feeding | WC | 183 | 280 | 19.91 | 0.000 |
| | PC | 280 | 351 | 7.76 | 0.005 |
| | SE | 230 | 394 | 42.59 | 0.000 |
| Washing | WC | 129 | 272 | 50.28 | 0.000 |
| | PC | 228 | 304 | 10.57 | 0.001 |
| | SE | 144 | 352 | 86.39 | 0.000 |
| Dressing | WC | 142 | 186 | 5.64 | 0.016 |
| | PC | 197 | 259 | 8.16 | 0.004 |
| | SE | 217 | 400 | 53.68 | 0.000 |
| Undressing | WC | 231 | 175 | 7.45 | 0.006 |
| | PC | 189 | 282 | 17.90 | 0.000 |
| | SE | 243 | 400 | 37.84 | 0.000 |
| Exercising | WC | 000 | 199 | 117.00 | 0.000 |
| | PC | 278 | 250 | 111.38 | 0.231 |
| | SE | 313 | 300 | 0.23 | 0.634 |
| Communication | | | | | |
| Patient | WC | 80 | 14 | 44.94 | 0.000 |
| | PC | 153 | 42 | 61.15 | 0.000 |
| | SE | 137 | 80 | 14.53 | 0.000 |
| Nurse | WC | 85 | 137 | 11.71 | 0.001 |
| | PC | 33 | 118 | 45.84 | 0.000 |
| | SE | 43 | 120 | 35.50 | 0.000 |

WC = wholly compensatory, PC = partly compensatory, SE = supportive–educative.

undressing activities for patients within each nursing system. The difference between wards in the quality of exercise activities for partly compensatory and supportive–educative patients was not significant. Many of the observations related to exercise were initiated by the patient, with the result that the more independent patients were able to perform this activity therapeutically. In White Ward a higher proportion of patients was dependent on staff for mobility activities, with the result that proportionally fewer exercise activities were performed. As far as the quality of communication between nurses and patients was concerned, there was more patient-initiated interaction in Brown Ward. Patients in partly compensatory and supportive–educative categories in Brown Ward were found to have fewer communication defects, e.g. fewer suffered from aphasia or deafness. Perhaps as a compensation for patients' limited communication ability, nurses in White Ward initiated significantly more conversation than did nursing staff in Brown Ward.

In order to describe the qualitative differences between observations in Brown and White Ward, particular patients experiences will be given to illustrate how patients self-care needs were met in each of the different nursing systems.

### Wholly compensatory patients

Each of the six patients in this category required regular and extensive nursing assistance in the performance of self-care activities. The majority of patients were immobile, mentally clouded, and had a range of communication difficulties such as asphasia, dysarthria and deafness. Despite such limitations, most of the elimination needs of patients in White Ward were met in a way that was described as moderately therapeutic (55.8% of activities were given a score of 3). In contrast, the majority of activities relating to patients' elimination needs in Brown Ward were minimally or non-therapeutic.

Nellie M, for example, a patient in Brown Ward for over 6 years, suffered from severe senile dementia, deafness and immobility. She was doubly incontinent and although her nursing care plan recommended that she be toiletted every 2 hours, this seldom occurred. Nellie spent most of her time in bed, where little attempt was made by nursing staff to control her bladder and bowel action.

Lizzie M in White Ward also suffered from severe senile dementia, was deaf and had poor vision. Staff usually got her up to sit in a geriatric chair just before breakfast and would bring her to the toilet. Lizzie was taken to the toilet after each meal and staff were encouraged to observe any restless behaviour, which might have been an indication of her need to eliminate. Although Lizzie was incontinent at times, nursing staff were observed making positive attempts to control bladder and bowel habits through a regular toilet regimen and observation of the patient for signs of restlessness or agitation.

Whereas Nellie M and Lizzie M had similar feeding requirements, the approaches adopted by staff in the two wards to meet their needs were quite distinct. Nellie was given breakfast in bed, which invariably consisted of porridge, tea and a piece of bread. A nurse would stand by her, giving her sips of porridge and tea. Lizzie, on the other hand, was usually up sitting in her geriatric chair for breakfast. A non-slip mat was placed on the detachable table in front of her and the nurse would ask her what she would like to eat. The nurse would the show Lizzie where her plate, spoon, tea and bread were by guiding her hand toward the implements. Although Lizzie was rather slow and spilled her food, she was still able to attempt to feed herself with assistance and encouragement from nursing staff.

Other patients in the wholly compensatory category were not quite as dependent on nursing staff, yet the amount of independence attained by patients in White Ward was significantly better. Florence B was a good example of an elderly female patient who had suffered a cerebrovascular accident some years earlier and had been left with extensive left-sided paralysis and severe aphasia. On White Ward, nursing staff tried to encourage her to be as independent as possible in her self-care activities. After being brought to the toilet, staff would put Florence into her geriatric chair, where they would proceed to dress her. She wore a complete set of undergarments and was consulted as to what she would like to wear each day. Although she could not express herself verbally, she would communicate her wishes by nodding or shaking her head and by squeezing the nurse's hand when she was particularly pleased about something. After she had been dressed, Florence was given a chance to wash her face and hands. A basin, her washbag and a towel were set on the table in front of her and she was left to spend some time fixing herself.

John A in Brown Ward also required help from nursing staff in dressing and washing activities. Although his vision was diminished, John was still mentally clear and able to communicate quite well with staff. He was very stiff and his immobility tended to dictate the level of nursing assistance provided in certain self-care activities. After breakfast in bed, which was often given to him by a nurse, John A would wait until someone came to attend to his elimination needs; he was often found to be incontinent and, after washing him, the nurse would proceed to dress him – trousers over pyjama bottoms, jumper or cardigan sometimes over pyjama top. His clothes were not his own and were often not the correct size. He would usually thank the nurse for dressing him and at the end of the activity, when he was set in his wheelchair, he was given a damp facecloth with which to rub his face.

Patients in this category received no exercise in Brown Ward and very little in White Ward. Rachel M, an elderly lady in White Ward who had right-sided weakness and suffered from senile dementia, was observed being walked to the day-room on a few occasions with the help of two nurses. This action had been taken in order to give Rachel practice in walking, although the staff involved in the activity often did not display depth of knowledge about how best to raise a dependent patient from a chair and how to support the patient when walking. Staff on Brown Ward did not seem to see the need to exercise such patients; they also seemed unaware of the need to provide patients in this category with a change of scenery or a feeling of independence, which could have been provided by taking them for a walk in a wheelchair.

Queenie S in Brown Ward was able to initiate and respond to verbal stimulation. She contributed to a substantial number of interactions initiated by patients in the communication section. In White Ward very few patients in this category were able to communicate verbally, Lizzie M and Florence B responding only to direct questioning from nursing staff.

## Partly compensatory patients

Four patients in White Ward were classed in the partly compensatory category, whereas two in Brown Ward came under this title. Patients' self-care abilities were limited in certain areas, but their self-care potential was such that improvement in function, with help and support from nursing staff, was considered a realistic goal. Patients in the partly compensatory category in both wards tended to spend most time on self-care needs, although the quality of the activities was found to differ significantly.

Patients' elimination needs were met more therapeutically in White Ward. Over 62% of observations were classed as moderately therapeutic (level 3), compared with 28% of observations in Brown Ward (see scores in table 34). Whereas just under 2% of observations associated with elimination activities were non-therapeutic in White Ward, 36% of observations in Brown Ward were non-therapeutic. Jack M's experiences in Brown Ward serve as an elucidating example of non-therapeutic nursing activity in careing for elimination needs in a patient in the partly compensatory category. Jack M's main problem was his immobility, caused by arthritis. Until his admission to hospital he had managed with assistance from his daughter and a home help who called in each morning to get him up. However, his circumstances changed when his daughter's support was reduced due to her husband's illness, leaving Jack M alone for a large part of the day. A fall precipitated Jack's hospital admission.

The aim of hospitalisation for Jack M was to assess his mobility and self-care potential, with a view to returning home with support from the home help. The nature and pattern of his incontinence was an important area of investigation, and the medical recommendation was that he be commenced on a habit retraining chart. The request, however, was not detailed in the patient's nursing care plan, nor was there any evidence that nursing staff were aware of the need to monitor his elimination pattern. Jack's limited mobility affected his independence in this area of self-care; very rarely were nursing staff seen to anticipate Jack's needs or assist him so that he could meet his elimination needs in privacy and with the optimal amount of independence. The result was that the majority of observations relating to Jack's elimination activities were poorly initiated and poorly effected, the outcome of which was minimally therapeutic for the patient.

In White Ward, Louisa B also had a problem with continence. This was linked with a diminished mental ability and mobility limitations. Whereas the medical goal was not as definite for Louisa, the nursing care goal had been quite clearly stated. A habit retraining chart had been commenced and was found to be filled in accurately each time Louisa went to the toilet or was incontinent. Nursing staff were all aware of the regimen and continued it when sister was off duty. Even though Louisa was often unable to recognise the need to eliminate, by observing her elimination pattern and, from that, by assessing bladder capacity and evacuation times, nursing staff were able to reduce her level of incontinence. Such elimination activities were seen as therapeutic.

The decision to serve breakfast in White Ward after patients had been allowed time to go to the toilet, and to get washed and dressed, guaranteed a much higher level of therapeutic activity than in Brown Ward. Like John A, Jack M (also in Brown Ward) was given breakfast in bed, the cantilever table often positioned at a height appropriate to facilitate easy manipulation of food. Margaret N's experience in White Ward was quite different. Described as a 'picky eater', whose favourite meal was breakfast, Margaret preferred a lightly boiled egg with brown bread and marmalade. This was provided for her each morning without any noticeable difficultly for staff. The other patients in White Ward were also given a choice, which included cooked breakfast, fruit juice, boiled eggs and toast. None of the patients in this category had difficulty in feeding themselves, despite a considerable level of mobility limitation. For each meal, they were positioned in such a way that they could manage their food with the minimum of assistance.

Washing and dressing activities were well underway in White Ward before breakfast was served. Sitting at their bedsides, patients were encouraged to dress themselves. By having her garments put out in sequence by nursing staff, Alice J, who suffered from senile dementia, was able to dress herself with supervision, whereas Betty K took great pride in being able to dress herself completely despite her hemiplegia: she only needed help with her shoes. In contrast, Jack M was dressed by a nurse, who began the activity while the patient was still sitting in bed. No attempt was made to encourage him to start dressing himself, as he was left in bed with the cotsides up until nursing staff came to attend him. On one occasion, Jack M was observed reaching over the cotside to his locker and poking out his shirt with the rounded end of his walking stick; he then proceeded to take off his pyjama jacket and put on his shirt. He buttoned up the shirt incorrectly, however, and was later reprimanded by the nurse for trying to do something that to her he was obviously incapable of doing.

Partly compensatory patients were generally involved in more exercise activities than were the wholly compensatory group. Although a medical goal for Jack M in Brown Ward was to improve mobilisation, very few attempts were made on the ward to achieve this. He was a difficult person to mobilise as he had one arthrosed knee joint and a rigidity that made attempts at helping him to stand more difficult. Things were not made any easier for nursing staff by sitting Jack in a low chair. This meant that he could give minimal assistance when nursing staff were trying to get him up. In contrast, staff in White Ward seemed to be more aware of the techniques involved in raising patients out of chairs and in guiding and supporting their mobility activities. For example, in addition to trying to improve Louisa B's elimination habits, an attempt was made to improve her walking ability. This plan was initiated by sister, transmitted to all staff and began with encouraging Louisa to stand upright for a few minutes at a time supported by two staff; it then progressed to the patient standing upright, supporting herself on a Zimmer frame. The next stage involved getting Louisa to take a few steps from her bedside to a chair in the ward. The distance was gradually increased, and practice was given each day, often linked with the patient's walk out to the toilet.

*Supportive–educative patients*
The third nursing category comprised three patients in Brown Ward and one in White Ward. The common characteristic of this group was that patient's self-care abilities were at a level that more often required only supervision and support from nursing staff rather than acting and doing for patients. Two of the patients, Martha O in Brown Ward and Sally S in White Ward, had similar self-care needs in that they were both physically quite independent but required a measure of support because of mental frailty. In contrast, Joseph D and Sam M (both also in Brown Ward) had a range of mobility and self-care limitations, but their potential for recovery was reckoned to be good. The nursing activity related to their care involved guiding, directing and providing support in order to enhance and develop their self-care potential.

Both Sally S and Martha O were independent in most self-care activities and were able to communicate their need for help to nursing staff. In consequence, both patients maintained a level of care that was therapeutic. The self-care activities of Joseph D and

Sam M, however, were found to be minimally therapeutic in the majority of situations. Both patients suffered from the routine approach to care at the beginning of the day, when ward staff attempted to meet patients' elimination needs, provide breakfast and wash and dress almost simultaneously within the first hour of coming on duty. Sam M's breakfast was served to him in bed. As the cotsides, which were still put up each evening, were seldom lowered for him at breakfast time, it meant that he often ate his food by lifting it from the cantilever table over the cotsides to his mouth. After breakfast he would sit and wait until a nurse came to bring him to the toilet or dress him. He made no attempt to dress himself, nor did nursing staff recognise the need to encourage him to practise skills that he had mastered in occupational therapy. One student nurse was observed trying to get him to dress himself one morning. However, rather than helping him with certain procedures, she chose to reprimand him by telling him that he was lazy and could dress himself perfectly well but was just not trying. This nurse left Sam trying to dress himself when another student, who had not been aware of the earlier conversation, came in and finished dressing him!

In Joseph D's case, dressing, washing and exercising were carried out by staff in a way that denied him the chance to help or assist in his own self-care activities. Joseph was able to walk without help in physiotherapy, yet in the ward he was wheeled to the toilet in a sanichair and was not encouraged to move around dependently in the ward. His continence problem had not been confronted by nursing staff until a considerable time after it had been noted in the medical chart that he should be commenced on a habit retraining chart. Feeding was also made difficult by the fact that he had poor vision and required to be given proper utensils and positioned in such a way that he could manage food easily. On the ward Joseph seemed to be very dependent on nursing staff, yet in physiotherapy his behaviour was very different: he talked more, he walked and he seemed more aware of the outside environment.

Thus, for patients in the supportive–educative category who could not articulate their needs or who were relearning motor and self-care skills, the nursing care in Brown Ward was minimally therapeutic. Nurses seemed to be least effective in helping patients in this category. Their lack of knowledge of patients' self-care abilities and self-care potential rendered their nursing

assistance quite insufficient to meet the particular needs of Sam M
and Joseph D. For Martha O and Sally S the inadequacies of
nursing activity were not as distinct, as both patients were able to
attend to their own self-care needs.

**Comments**

The results of the comparative case study have shown a distinct
variation in the quality of nursing care provided to patients in
Brown and White Ward. Whereas the amount of time patients
spent in self-care activities did not differ significantly, the quality
of the activities in terms of the nurse's therapeutic contribution
and the patient's outcome did vary in each of the three nursing
systems.

The nurse's contribution to patient care in the wholly compensatory category comprised acting on behalf of and doing for the
patient. In Brown Ward such activity took a routine, non-
personalised approach to meeting patients' self-care needs. Little
consideration was given to patients' self-care abilities or potential.
Feeding, washing, dressing and meeting elimination needs were
approached in a collective manner, without consideration of
patients' individual requests or preferences. In White Ward,
nursing activity was more patient-oriented. Whereas nurses still
acted on patients' behalf, they considered each patient's self-care
ability and potential. They also made use of the environment so
that it could provide patients with more independence; they
safeguarded patients' right to choose and there was also more
personal contact between staff and patients.

For patients in the partly compensatory category, staff in White
Ward aimed to provide an environment that was conducive to
maintaining and developing independence and self-care skills.
This was seen in the way in which patients were positioned for
meals and in the way washing and dressing activities were
enhanced by careful positioning. Patients in this category were
also given the opportunity of choosing what they would eat, what
they would wear and when they would perform certain activities.
Nursing staff also provided more direct support by guiding and
helping patients to master certain self-care skills. Nursing activity
for this category in Brown Ward tended to concentrate on the
acting and doing roles of the nurse. Patients' levels of self-care
were not improved by careful use of the environment, nor did

nurses seem to be aware of their role as supporters, guides and teachers of patients. Patients were given little choice in what happened to them, not only in the main self-care activities but also in their choice of whom they sat beside, where they sat and when they went to bed.

Nursing action in the supportive–educative category also differed between wards. Staff in Brown Ward continued to approach their work from the point of view of acting and doing for patients rather than using the range of assisting techniques available to them. Whereas patients in this category were most independent in areas of self-care, they were still treated in the same 'batch' manner. Staff in White Ward provided more differentiated care and ensured that patients in the supportive–educative category were allowed time to perform their own self-care activities. The environment was used in such a way that it stimulated independence, and both staff and patients were cognisant of the goals of self-care toward which they were working.

Staff performance and patient experiences were thought to be related to the ward sister's level of therapeutic awareness of her nursing function. Thus, Sister White, who had a high TNF score, was able to provide a higher quality of care by motivating and guiding her staff to consider patients' individual needs and by encouraging them to provide the most appropriate sort of nursing assistance from the range of identifiable helping activities. Sister Brown and her team provided care that was less therapeutic or at a lower standard because she was not aware of her therapeutic nursing function. This resulted in a poorly differentiated work role for staff, poor identification of patients' individual needs and a routine approach to nursing care.

Sister White's positive therapeutic nursing function manifested itself in the way she organised nursing activity. She recognised the importance of obtaining detailed assessments of patients' self-care abilities and used this information to organise and plan nursing care. Staff were kept aware of patients' individual needs and were encouraged to use a range of skills. Routines were also geared to patients' needs. Breakfast, for example, was served at 9.00 a.m. to ensure the patients had time to get up and prepare themselves for the first meal of the day. Sister White also saw her caring role as extending to counselling both patients and relatives. She delegated responsibility and included nursing auxiliaries in report sessions. She also spent time teaching student nurses and auxiliaries how to perform such activities as lifting patients and transferring them from chairs to commodes; she encouraged staff to use afternoons as a time for socialising with patients, getting to know them and stimulating them by organising sherry parties and sing-songs or by playing games.

Sister Brown's poor perception of her therapeutic nursing function was reflected in the diffuse goal content for patient care. The nursing goal for most patients seemed to be linked to getting through the work. Nursing activity in consequence involved getting patients up, washed, dressed and fed as quickly as possible so that the more 'important' work of rehabilitation could commence. Work was not organised as it was not seen to vary – the routine was always the same. This led to some staff complaining that they did not need training to do the work they were doing, whereas others felt adrift because they did not know what patients could or could not do for themselves. The result was that neither patients' self-care needs nor their self-care potential were identified, and nursing care was routinised and meaning- less. Nurses' skill repertoire was limited to acting and doing for patients and, even at this level, staff were not encouraged to use the environment as a therapeutic tool or to maintain environmental conditions that would protect and support normal function. Nursing knowledge of patients' personal needs was minimal, a reflection of the lack of involvement that Sister Brown had with patients' emotional reactions and their adjustment to hospitalisation and increased dependence.

Outcomes for patients being cared for in a ward where staff had a poor perception of their therapeutic nursing function were loss of dignity, diminution of the right to make choices, minimal independence and little regard for patients' personal feelings and emotions. Some staff were unhappy about the care they gave, feeling frustrated by the lack of information and the rigid routine, yet feeling powerless to change it. Other staff in the ward did not see anything wrong with the care they provided, given the poor staff numbers and the physically demanding nature of the job.

Thus, it would appear that a significant factor that influenced the standard of patient care was the ward sister's awareness of her therapeutic nursing function. This conclusion was reached by consideration of the results obtained from comparing the quantity and quality of nursing care given to patients in two ward environments, which were matched for a range of extraneous variables such as medical and paramedical input, the level of ancillary services and nursing management policy. The main difference was that the sister in Brown Ward had a low TNF score and the sister in White Ward had a high TNF score.

In order to test the conclusion, a further study was carried out in a ward where the ward sister's TNF score matched that of Sister Brown, but where extraneous variables differed. The purpose of this study was to compare the quantity and quality of nursing care on the two wards under the influence of different extraneous variables but where the ward sister's approach was considered to be similar. If extraneous variables had a significant influence on nursing care, in a ward environment like Red Ward, where both medical and paramedical influence was more direct, one would expect nursing staff to hold a more positive and therapeutic approach to care. If the ward sister's perception of her work role was more influential on staff and on the way they went about their work, one would expect to find a less therapeutic approach to care, despite the input from medical and paramedical facilities.

**Testing the finding**

Red Ward was situated on the upper floor of a modern, purpose-built geriatric unit on the site of a large general hospital. It had not been included in the social survey; another ward in the building had been studied, and the intention had been to use that ward in the comparative analysis. However, when the researcher came to undertake the study, the ward sister in the original ward had changed, and another ward had to be found. The sister in a neighbouring ward (Red Ward) was approached and, being willing to participate, was asked to complete a staff questionnaire. She was found to have a TNF score of 75.

The ward differed from Brown and White Wards in its layout, the standard of its facilities, the approach that the medical personnel took to patient care and the part that paramedical workers played in the provision of patient care. Red Ward was L-shaped, with capacity for 36 patients; it had a ward profile score of 76, with toilet, day-room and storage facilities all in the 'good' category. It was well supplied with furniture and equipment, and ancillary services were provided by the main hospital departments. All types of geriatric patient were admitted to the ward, from acute and assessment patients to rehabilitation and continuing care patients. The medical approach to treatment was to ensure a mix of patient types on each of the four geriatric wards in the unit, in the belief that such a mix was good for staff morale and patient care. The geriatric medical model, with its orientation towards diagnosis, assessment, rehabilitation and cure, was implicit in the approach that consultants adopted to interaction with patients and other members of the multidisciplinary team. The number of admissions and discharges was much greater than for either Brown and White Ward, Red Ward being seen more as an acute treatment environment than as a continuing care setting.

Paramedical input to patient care was noticeably increased, with the large physio- and occupational therapy departments servicing each of the four wards in the unit. The paramedical workers had a policy of treating both rehabilitation and continuing care patients. Each ward had its own physiotherapist and occupational therapist, whose responsibility it was to come to the ward and treat those patients who did not attend for treatment in either department. It was also seen as a way of ensuring that nursing staff on the ward were kept informed of patient progress in physio- and occupational therapy. There was also a full-time art therapist and a handicraft instructor in the occupational therapy department. In general, the atmosphere in the unit was one of intense activity, with paramedical departments servicing not only ward patients but also large numbers of day hospital patients.

Whereas the range of extraneous variables was quite distinct from those of White and Brown Ward, the sister's TNF score on Red Ward was similar to that of Sister Brown. From her TNF indicator responses, the sister in Red Ward appeared to have a poorly differentiated concept of geriatric care. Her management approach to nursing care seemed to be routine-oriented. She did not insist on detailed nursing assessment of patients' needs, nor was specific information on patients' self-care abilities or potential gathered. A work-list was made out each morning, which allocated groups of staff to perform certain duties. Despite the considerable contact with paramedical staff, the sister displayed a limited understanding of the nursing contribution to the rehabilitation of patients. She described rehabilitation in very much medically related terms, rehabilitation including those ranges of activities that are performed by the physiotherapist and occupational therapist in order to retrain the patient in self-care skills, with the goal of complete recovery and discharge.

The sister's TNF indicator results were somewhat atypical give her age, academic qualifications and environmental conditions. However, interviews with nursing staff and with the sister herself reinforced the findings of the TNF indicator. As in Brown and White Ward, the nursing staff in Red Ward were given the opportunity to comment on aspects of their work. The ward team comprised three SRNs, seven SENs, four second-year student nurses and two full-time nursing auxiliaries. In general, the SRNs reflected the sister's approach to care, identifying as important such areas as meeting patients' basic needs and keeping them clean and tidy. More emphasis was put on carrying out medical prescriptions and treating acutely ill patients, a reflection of the fact that Red Ward admitted a high proportion of such patients. None of the staff nurses felt that more information should be obtained from patients, and they seemed to be happy with the way work was organised on the ward.

The SENs in Red Ward, however, did not reflect the same measure of satisfaction with the way work was organised. The majority felt that the nursing care plans did not provide them with enough information about patients, nor were they given any detailed information at report times. They were not aware of the treatment that patients received at physio- and occupational therapy. One SEN suggested that a sheet documenting all patients' problems and ways of treating them should be available to staff on the ward. SENs also mentioned their feelings of frustration at not being able to develop a wider range of skills. They felt that they were given the more 'routine' jobs, whereas SRNs were given more 'interesting' jobs, such as giving out medicines and being in charge of the ward. Although they would have liked more information on patients' needs, they continued to see their main role as the provision of basic nursing care. In this they were in accord with the ward sister.

Student nurses in Red Ward described geriatric nursing as hard work but enjoyable. As far as obtaining information on individual patients was concerned, they felt it was up to each one of them to use their own initiative to find out as much as they could. They agreed that there was no organised system of communicating information about patients on the ward and that it was difficult to know what patients could and could not do for themselves.

Both nursing auxiliaries were satisfied with their work; neither

| Patient | Category | Observation of therapeutic nursing action |
|---|---|---|
| Margaret W | Wholly compensatory | *Elimination needs*<br>1. Do staff meet patient's request for toilet promptly?<br>2. Is patient prevented from becoming constipated? |

*Diagnosis*
Rheumatoid arthritis
Partial vision

*Feeding*
1. Is patient given a choice of food?
2. Is environment used therapeutically?
3. Are appropriate aids and appliances used?
4. Are mealtimes socially stimulating?

*Self-care requirements*
● Needs to be washed and dressed
● Assistance with elimination
● Prone to constipation
● Mobility limitation – dependent on staff

*Washing, dressing, undressing*
1. Does patient have a choice in what she wears?
2. What is the level of interaction between patient and nurse?
3. Are patient's privacy and dignity maintained?

*Self-care potential*
● Able to feed self with adequate positioning in geriatric chair and provision of special cutlery
● Mentally alert, requires stimulation

*Exercising*
1. Does patient receive passive exercise?
2. Do paramedical and nursing staff have an activity plan for patient?

*Communication*
1. Do staff initiate general conversation?

---

| Patient | Category | Observation of therapeutic nursing action |
|---|---|---|
| Mary W | Partly compensatory | *Elimination needs*<br>1. Is patient given assistance in going to toilet?<br>2. Is she encouraged to perform activity independently? |

*Diagnosis*
Right hemiplegia
Expressive aphasia

*Feeding*
1. Is patient given a choice of food?
2. Is environment used therapeutically?
3. Are mealtimes used as a source of increased social stimulation?

*Self-care requirements*
● Requires support and assistance in washing and dressing activities
● Can go to toilet by self
● Wears plastazole boot and caliper on right leg. Can stand with help and walk by self using tripod
● Requires social stimulation and contact with others as is prone to depression

*Washing, dressing, undressing*
1. Are dressing skills taught by occupational therapist and reinforced by nursing assistance?
2. Is patient encouraged to perform these activities independently?
3. Is environment used therapeutically?

*Exercising*
1. Is patient encouraged to walk and practise right arm exercises?
2. Do staff advise patient in correct way to rise and sit down in chair?

**Self-care potential**
● Aim is independence in all self-care activities with discharge to residential accommodation

*Communication*
1. Do staff make an effort to involve patient in activities in the ward?

**Figure 12**  Nursing care plans and observation of therapeutic content of self-care activities

seemed to notice the lack of detailed information about patients, feeling secure in their routine approach to patient care.

Thus, as far as the interviews showed, staff reflected the same routine approach to patient care as had been manifested by the sister. Her main concern seemed to be in ensuring that acutely ill patients were cared for and that medical regimens were carried out. The SRNs tended to act as deputies for the sister, not getting involved with patient care, whereas the SENs and student nurses were in most frequent and intimate contact with patients.

The methods used to observe patients' self-care activity and nursing action were similar to the techniques employed in Brown and White Ward. Eight patients, representative of the total ward population, were chosen and divided into the three main nursing systems. During the observation period the number of patients in Red Ward dropped from 36 to 22. The ward was not admitting new patients, with the result that proportionately more continuing care and rehabilitation patients were found on the ward. This resulted in three patients in the study belonging to the wholly compensatory group, four to the partly compensatory group and one to the supportive–educative group (see appendix VIIIc in Kitson, 1984). Patients' nursing care plans were consulted, after which intermittent, non-participant observation of the eight patients began.

Nursing information on patients' self-care requirements, self-care ability and potential was found to be vague and inadequate. Nursing directions consisted of short statements on the patients' need for assistance in each of the main self-care areas. There was no detailed information about patients' mental and social ability and no direct assessment of their mobility limitations, nor was there any information about patients' likes and dislikes. More relevant and up-to-date information regarding patients' mobility and functional ability levels was found in medical and paramedical notes, and from this source the researcher was able to build up a picture of the self-care needs and potential of each of the patients being studied. Table 35 gives an example of the way in which patient information was used to guide the assessment of the therapeutic content of observations.

## Findings – comparison of Brown, White and Red Wards
Patients in Red Ward were found to spend significantly more time in contact with other members of the multidisciplinary team,

**Table 35**   Percentage of time spent in contact with members of multidisciplinary team

| | Total | | | Wholly compensatory | | | Partly compensatory | | | Supportive– educative | | |
|---|---|---|---|---|---|---|---|---|---|---|---|---|
| | B | W | R | B | W | R | B | W | R | B | W | R |
| Doctors | 0.1 | 0.1 | 0.1 | 0.0 | 0.1 | 0.0 | 0.3 | 0.0 | 0.1 | 0.1 | 0.1 | 0.0 |
| Physiotherapists | 2.3 | 2.0 | 4.2 | 0.0 | 1.3 | 5.2 | 2.4 | 1.9 | 2.5 | 4.3 | 5.0 | 7.5 |
| Occupational therapists | 1.1 | 0.3 | 3.4 | 0.0 | 0.0 | 4.5 | 4.4 | 0.4 | 1.3 | 0.2 | 0.0 | 8.1 |
| Others (art therapists) | 1.7 | 0.6 | 5.1 | 0.2 | 0.1 | 11.5 | 1.3 | 0.9 | 0.5 | 0.5 | 0.2 | 3.9 |
| Visitors | 3.1 | 4.1 | 3.3 | 3.8 | 2.8 | 5.1 | 2.3 | 5.7 | 2.1 | 2.9 | 1.5 | 2.3 |
| *Total* | 8.3 | 7.1 | 16.1 | 4.0 | 4.3 | 26.3 | 10.7 | 8.9 | 6.5 | 8.0 | 6.8 | 21.8 |

B = Brown Ward, W = White Ward, R = Red Ward.

particularly physiotherapists, occupational therapists and art therapists (table 35).

Interestingly, patients in the partly compensatory category in Red Ward had a low level of paramedical involvement (6.5%). This may be explained by the fact that two of the four patients in this category refused to go to physiotherapy or occupational therapy. The policy adopted by paramedical staff connected with Red Ward was to provide as much stimulation and therapy for wholly compensatory patients as for the more rehabilitable partly compensatory and supportive–educative patients.

Whereas more time was spent with paramedical staff, contact with medical personnel was as infrequent for patients on Red Ward as for patients on Brown and White Ward. The amount of time devoted to self-care activities on Red Ward was similar to that on Brown and White Ward (table 36). Wholly compensatory patients, however, spent less time on their self-care activities, whereas patients in the supportive–educative group in Red Ward spent most time in the performance of these activities.

There was no significant difference between wards as to any of the quantity scores. In terms of patient self-care activities, therefore, staff seemed to devote the same proportion of time to meeting patients' needs. This is interesting given the fact that White Ward had the lowest number of staff working on the ward each day whereas Red Ward had most staff on each duty shift. The median number of nurses on duty in White Ward was seven in the morning shift, five in the afternoon shift and four in the evening

**Table 36** Percentage of time spent in self-care activities in Brown, White and Red Wards

| Activity | Total | | | Wholly compensatory | | | Partly compensatory | | | Supportive – educative | | |
|---|---|---|---|---|---|---|---|---|---|---|---|---|
| | B | W | R | B | W | R | B | W | R | B | W | R |
| Elimination | 3.3 | 4.6 | 3.0 | 2.9 | 4.3 | 2.6 | 5.6 | 5.3 | 3.0 | 2.2 | 2.5 | 4.4 |
| Feeding | 8.1 | 8.2 | 6.5 | 7.9 | 8.8 | 6.5 | 7.2 | 7.8 | 6.2 | 8.8 | 8.0 | 7.4 |
| Drinking | 2.6 | 2.4 | 2.4 | 2.5 | 2.3 | 2.2 | 2.6 | 3.0 | 2.1 | 2.8 | 2.9 | 1.8 |
| Washing | 1.5 | 1.9 | 1.8 | 2.1 | 2.2 | 2.0 | 1.5 | 1.5 | 1.4 | 1.0 | 2.5 | 3.0 |
| Bathing | 0.3 | 0.3 | 0.2 | 0.1 | 0.2 | 0.2 | 0.1 | 0.5 | 0.3 | 0.6 | 0.2 | 0.1 |
| Dressing | 1.5 | 1.4 | 1.5 | 1.1 | 0.8 | 1.3 | 1.6 | 1.2 | 1.4 | 1.8 | 3.8 | 3.7 |
| Undressing | 1.1 | 1.4 | 1.3 | 1.1 | 1.3 | 0.8 | 1.1 | 1.2 | 1.3 | 1.1 | 2.3 | 2.0 |
| Exercising | 1.7 | 1.8 | 4.0 | 0.0 | 0.7 | 0.0 | 2.2 | 2.1 | 6.0 | 3.0 | 4.3 | 8.0 |
| Communicating | 1.7 | 3.0 | 2.3 | 1.4 | 2.2 | 2.1 | 2.9 | 3.4 | 2.7 | 1.3 | 3.0 | 1.8 |
| *Total* | 21.8 | 25.0 | 23.0 | 19.1 | 22.8 | 17.7 | 24.8 | 26.0 | 24.4 | 22.6 | 29.5 | 32.2 |

B = Brown Ward, W = White Ward, R = Red Ward.

**Table 37** Therapeutic content of self-care activities – summary scores
**a.** Comparison of Brown Ward and White Ward (low TNF score v. high TNF score)

| Activity | Brown Ward | White Ward | $\chi^2$ | $p$ |
|---|---|---|---|---|
| Elimination | 202 | 266 | 8.48 | 0.00 |
| Feeding | 224 | 326 | 27.62 | 0.00 |
| Washing | 156 | 253 | 22.53 | 0.00 |
| Dressing | 190 | 241 | 20.79 | 0.00 |
| Undressing | 203 | 259 | 6.57 | 0.01 |
| Exercising | 302 | 332 | 1.3265 | 0.24 |
| Communication | | | | |
| Patient | 128 | 39 | 46.37 | 0.00 |
| Nurse | 51 | 123 | 28.971 | 0.00 |

**b.** Comparison of Brown Ward and Red Ward (low TNF score v. low TNF score, difference in environmental conditions)

| Activity | Brown Ward | Red Ward | $\chi^2$ | $p$ |
|---|---|---|---|---|
| Elimination | 202 | 222 | 0.85 | 0.64 |
| Feeding | 224 | 252 | 4.844 | 0.03 |
| Washing | 156 | 174 | 0.875 | 0.67 |
| Dressing | 190 | 214 | 1.309 | 0.25 |
| Undressing | 203 | 233 | 0.161 | 1.93 |
| Exercising | 302 | 287 | 0.333 | 0.57 |
| Communication | | | | |
| Patient | 128 | 39 | 46.3711 | 0.00 |
| Nurse | 51 | 123 | 28.9711 | 0.00 |

shift; for Brown Ward the figures were eight or nine, seven and four or five, and for Red Ward ten, seven and five respectively. The large number of staff in Red Ward may explain why feeding activities were performed more quickly, in that more nursing staff were available to assist patients.

When the quality of nursing action was studied, a number of more distinct variations occurred between Brown and Red Ward and White and Red Ward. Using the same scaling method (see table 33) overall figures for the therapeutic content of self-care activities were compiled for all patients in Red Ward and then for patients in their separate nursing systems. Whereas the quality of nursing action was significantly different between Brown and White Ward, fewer of the results between Brown and Red Ward differed significantly (table 37). This led to the conclusion that the quality of care in Brown and Red Ward was similar, whereas the quality of care in White Ward was significantly better than both of these. Figures 13–16 below show the similarities and differences between the therapeutic content of nurse activity in patient care outcomes in each of the three wards.

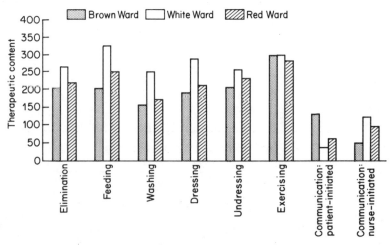

**Figure 13**   Effect of therapeutic content of nurse activity on patient outcomes – total patient population

In the wholly compensatory category (figure 14) the majority of self-care activities were performed in the most therapeutic way in White Ward. Such patients in White Ward were the only ones in that group to be exercised by nursing staff, and the level of nurse-initiated conversation was also highest in White Ward. Although patients in the partly compensatory category (figure 15) generally had a better therapeutic content in self-care activities, White Ward still provided the best care. Red Ward was found to be poorest in certain areas, particularly in feeding and washing activities. Exercise activities were slightly better in Brown and Red Ward than in White Ward. This could have been a reflection of the 'rehabiliation' orientation of Brown and Red Ward as opposed to White Ward's 'continuing care' label. Communication patterns tended to be similar in White and Red Ward, with nurses initiating most of the interactions.

Interpretation of the results for supportive–educative patients (figure 16) must take into consideration the fact that only one patient in White and Red Ward was observed, compared to three patients in Brown Ward. However, it was felt that the total number of observations (840) per patient was sufficient to enable an accurate judgment on the therapeutic content of the activity being performed to be made. Again, White Ward was found to provide the best quality of care, although this time Red Ward activity more closely resembled White Ward than Brown Ward. The improved care for supportive–educative patients was thought

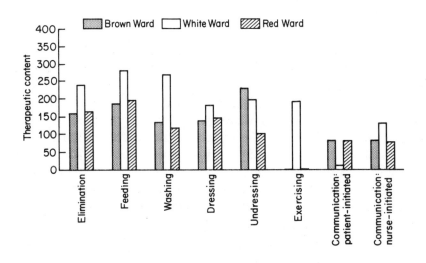

**Figure 14** Wholly compensatory patients

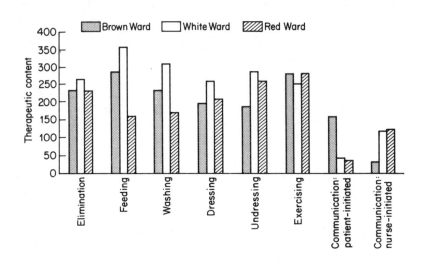

**Figure 15**  Partly compensatory patients

to reflect the greater orientation in Red Ward to the needs of rehabilitation patients, the increased contact of paramedical workers and the improved ward facilities. However, the high levels of therapeutic content for White Ward still demonstrated the central contribution of nursing staff in the provision of quality of care.

## Comments

Observation of patients' self-care activity on Red Ward was undertaken to ascertain whether or not variables such as the ward layout, the level of paramedical support and medical policies had any effect on the therapeutic content of nursing activity in meeting patients' self-care requirements. The findings suggest that such extraneous variables have less effect on the outcome than does the ward sister's awareness of her therapeutic nursing function. In order to reinforce this conclusion, several of the variables have been documented in more detail to show how staff reacted to such improvements in their ward environment. These include the use of improved toilet and day-room facilities and the effect of increased paramedical coverge on nursing activity.

*Toilet facilities.*   Red Ward had a total of six toilet facilities: two large toilet areas of 60 ft² (5.60 m²); three medium-sized areas of 28 ft$^2$ (2.6 m$^2$) and one small facility of 26 ft$^2$ (2 m$^2$). Four of the toilet areas were situated close to the large day-room, with the two other facilities adjacent to the smaller sitting area in another part of the ward. The large toilet facilities had been designed to accommodate a chairfast patient and two assistants. The medium-sized toilet areas were not sufficiently large to take a geriatric chair; often nurses were seen positioning the chair in the open doorway and then transferring the patient from the chair to the toilet seat. Medium-sized facilities were best suited to semi-ambulant patients who could manage with a Zimmer frame or required the assistance of one nurse. The small toilet area best served those ambulant patients with minimal mobility and self-care limitations.

Each of the toilet areas in Red Ward was larger and of a better design than the facilities in either Brown or White Ward, yet use of the facilities was generally not therapeutic to patient outcomes. For example, Henry C, an immobile, incontinent patient in the wholly compensatory category, was seldom observed being taken to the toilet despite the fact that facilities existed in which he could be transferred from his geriatric chair to the toilet in privacy and with minimal difficulty for staff. Instead, Henry was allowed to remain doubly incontinent, staff considering the change of clothing after mealtimes less bothersome than trying to retrain his bladder and bowel habits. Staff often used the medium-sized toilet

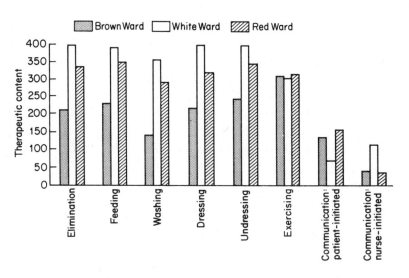

**Figure 16** Supportive–educative patients

facilities for chairfast patients, whereas other, more mobile patients used the large facilities. This meant that for the more dependent patients privacy was eroded and toiletting activities rendered more difficult for staff.

Toilet facilities were more therapeutically used by patients in the partly compensatory and supportive–educative categories in Red Ward. Mary W, for example, was able to walk to the toilet using a tripod. She then had sufficient space in one of the medium-sized toilet facilities to manoeuvre herself plus tripod to enable her to meet her elimination needs independently. Rose G was also able to achieve independence in elimination needs by being provided with a raised toilet seat. She was then able to pull herself up off the toilet, supporting herself with two handrails, one on either side of the toilet.

Improved toilet facilities, however, did not augment the therapeutic content of Robert R's elimination activities. Robert suffered from senile dementia and incontinence. His continence problem was also causing a range of other problems, in that Robert's elimination habits were less than socially acceptable. It was recommended that his elimination pattern be recorded on a habit retraining chart, with a view to modifying his behaviour and improving continence. Nursing staff, however, did not seem to be aware of Robert's particular problems and were seldom seen assisting or encouraging him to use toilet facilities at regular intervals. Consequently, Robert's elimination pattern did not improve, and on occasions he was prevented from attending physio- and occupational therapy because of his inability to control elimination. Nursing staff did not seem to be aware of the fact that they had failed to orientate Robert or to get him used to eliminating after mealtimes or at other set times. Thus, whereas the improved facilities helped certain patients, those who were most dependent on nursing staff for ensuring therapeutic activity did not benefit from the improved facilities in the ward. The deficit appeared to result from the nurse's orientation and approach to her activity.

*Day-room facilities.* Red Ward had two day-rooms; the larger day-room space of over 1000 ft² (93 m²) was used for most patients on the ward, whereas the smaller space of 248 ft² (23 m²) provided a sitting area for the more confused or disruptive patients. The large day-room was the centre of activity for the whole ward. Easily accessible to both staff and patients, it was convenient for toilet areas and ward bays. Patients also ate lunch and tea in the day-room, grouped around dining tables. For those patients who were mentally alert and able to communicate, the day-room was a source of social stimulation. However, for patients like Mary W, who suffered from severe expressive aphasia, the day-room was as isolated, in terms of contact with other patients and nursing staff, as sitting alone in the ward bay. Mary W used to sit by herself each day in the day-room; she had her meals in the same place and was rarely seen communicating with either patients or staff. Although in Mary's medical notes it was recommended that nursing staff should make an effort to involve her in social interaction, staff did not appear to perceive having to sit down and talk with Mary as part of their job.

Thus, the improved facilities were seen to increase social interaction of certain patients, particularly the more vocal and alert, whereas for patients who required support and encouragement from nursing staff to communicate and interact more fully, the day-room did not provide any great benefit. Again, the therapeutic content of the activity seemed to rest with the nurse's ability to perceive and meet patients' particular self-care requirements.

*Paramedical coverage.* The additional support provided by paramedical staff was found to have a significant effect on the amoung of time that patients in Red Ward spent in contact with members of the multidisciplinary team. This was particularly evident for wholly compensatory patients. Physio- and occupational therapists provided both rehabilitative and maintenance therapy for all patients in the geriatric ward. Thus, patients in Red Ward in the so-called medically designated continuing care category were treated by therapists, whereas in Brown and White Wards little paramedical time was devoted to this group. The additional stimulation was seen as therapeutic for patients, although the benefits accrued in the departments were not found to be carried over into the ward situation. For example, Sarah F was able to perform a range of manipulative skills in occupational therapy, whereas on the ward she was often fed by nursing staff. The self-care abilities that had been identified in occupational therapy seemed to be neither recognised nor utilised in the ward setting. Patients were allowed to choose whether they attended physio- or occupational therapy, as evidenced by the fact that two patients from the partly compensatory group chose not to attend. A physiotherapist would come to see such patients in the ward and practise walking or other mobility activities with them. For example, Mary W had decided not to attend physiotherapy, and a therapist came to see her on the ward, where she watched Mary getting up from her chair and encouraged her in the correct use of her tripod and in getting up from and sitting down in her chair. Although the physiotherapist was observed teaching the patient, she did not involve staff in explaining how best to manoeuvre patients. The result was that when nursing staff were responsible for helping Mary out of her chair and setting her down, practices that the physiotherapist had vetoed were being performed by nursing staff.

Thus, the benefits of the specialist skills of the therapists did not appear to be successfully integrated into the self-care activities performed by nurses and patients on the ward. Paramedical and nursing staff seemed to share neither information on patients nor ways in which either party could have ensured a more therapeutic approach to care. The outcome was that good practices, which were being encouraged by paramedical workers, were not being reinforced by nursing staff because of the lack of awareness of the techniques used and, perhaps more significantly, because nursing staff had not assessed the individual self-care requirements of their patients.

Improved ward facilities and a more comprehensive and progressive paramedical contribution to patient care was thought to have some effect on the overall therapeutic content of patient care in the partly compensatory and supportive–educative categories in Red Ward. For patients in the wholly compensatory category, any benefit provided by the environment would be through the nurse's contribution to patient care. Thus in White Ward, where nursing staff were most aware of their therapeutic nursing function, patient care was improved in all areas of self-care activity. In Brown Ward, where environmental and para-medical input was similar to that of White Ward, but where nursing staff had a poor perception of their therapeutic nursing function, patient care was found to be of a lower standard. The therapeutic content of nursing activity in Red Ward was found to be influenced more by the nursing staff's poor perception of their therapeutic nursing function than by the effect of a range of external factors, particularly for patients who were most dependent on nursing staff to meet their self-care activities. This leads to the conclusion that it is the nurse's, and more specifically the ward sister's awareness of her therapeutic nursing function that determines the therapeutic content of care on the ward.

## Summary

The object of the case study was to determine whether or not the TNF indicator was a sensitive measure of the nurse's therapeutic activity in the ward situation and to investigate the effect of such factors as the influence of medical and paramedical workers and the ward environment on the quantity and quality of nursing care. This was done by observing nursing activity on three wards, which varied in the ward sister's TNF level and in certain extraneous variables. The results showed that none of the extraneous variables described above had as important an effect on the quality of care as did the ward sister's own perception of nursing. The ward sister's approach to nursing was measured by her TNF score, which was seen as a direct reflection of her acceptance of her *caring* role.

Three ward environments were used to test the effect of such variables on the quantity and quality of patient care. Although Brown and White Wards were matched in ward environment, medical and paramedical coverage, there was a significant difference between the therapeutic content of patients' self-care activities. This variation reflected the position of each ward sister on the TNF indicator scale, less therapeutic care linked with the low TNF scoring ward sister and more therapeutic care being found in the high scoring TNF sister's ward. When the quality of care was measured in two wards (Brown and Red), where sisters had low TNF scores but ward environment, medical and paramedical input differed, the therapeutic content of patients' self-care activities did not differ significantly.

A number of other interesting points emerged in the study. First, the amount of time spent in self-care activities did not differ significantly in any of the three wards, regardless of the variation in staffing levels and in the standard of ward facilities. Second, in Red Ward it was the wholly compensatory patients who fared worst in terms of self-care activities, whereas for partly compensatory and supportive–educative patients the increased paramedical involvement and a better ward environment had the effect of improving the therapeutic content of the majority of their self-care activities. In Brown Ward, where little emphasis was put on paramedical input or on the maintenance of patients' self-care abilities, partly compensatory and supportive—educative patients experienced significantly poorer care than did patients in either Red or White Ward. Each category of patient in White Ward received care that was therapeutic. For wholly compensatory patients in particular, the therapeutic content of self-care activities was significantly better. Finally, these observations of the variations within and between wards led to the conclusion that it was the sister's understanding of her caring role, realised by the nursing staff, that determined the therapeutic content of the majority of patient activities.

In addition to testing the validity of the TNF indicator, the case study was also used to develop and test a quality of care indicator, the TNF Matrix. The TNF Matrix was based on the main theoretical concepts of the nursing theory and used assessments of patients' self-care potential and need for nursing to evaluate the therapeutic content of nursing action and patients' self-care activities. The strength of the matrix as a quality of care indicator was seen to lie in its ability to consider a range of factors in coming to a decision about the quality of care. For example, the therapeutic content of an activity was judged on how the nurse used her knowledge of patients' self-care requirements to organise the most appropriate care, which would ensure optimal independence in self-care activities. Observation of patients' elimination and feeding self-care activities, in particular, identified the therapeutic content of patients' activities and the extent to which nursing staff were aware of their therapeutic contribution to patient care.

# 7 Summary and conclusions

The study began with a consideration of the concept of care and the nurse's contribution to the care of the hospitalised elderly. Although at the outset it may have seemed a straightforward task, adequate explanation of these areas soon involved the development of a theoretical framework, based on the concept of self-care, in order to explain the nurse's role in the provision of care.

The development of a theoretical framework for geriatric nursing was the first step taken toward identifying the dimensions of nursing's caring role. Commencing with the guidelines laid down by Norton et al (1962), the theoretical framework for geriatric nursing was augmented by relevant concepts from Orem's (1980) self-care theory and fashioned by Dickoff et al's (1968) construction guide for theories in nursing. The emerging nursing theory emphasised both the need for the patient to be maintained in a state of optimal self-care and independence, and the need to recognise the dynamic nature of the nurse's contribution to the achievement of such a goal. In terms of her caring role, the nurse was seen as having to combine a rational and pragmatic approach to the assessment of patients' self-care requirements with planning and organising individualised patient care. Her caring role also comprised more emotional and personal aspects, which enabled her to comfort and support the patient.

The successful merging of this range of skills, which was seen as fundamental to care, was termed the nurse's therapeutic function. A measurement instrument, called the TNF indicator, was constructed in order to see whether this collection of attributes existed and whether it was an accurate representation of the skills that were characteristic of nurses who provided more patient-centred care. Based on the theoretical concepts already developed, the TNF

217

indicator was used to distinguish those sisters in geriatric wards who had a positive concept of their caring role (characterised by a high score on the TNF indicator scale) from those sisters who had little understanding of the dimensions of their caring role (characterised by a low score on the TNF indicator scale).

The development of the TNF indicator, through the identification and operationalisation of concepts from the theoretical framework, ensured a measure of content validity for the instrument. Steps toward ensuring the instrument's reliability involved testing the TNF indicator on a randomly selected, representative sample of sisters in geriatric wards in Northern Ireland. Ward sisters came from a variety of backgrounds, worked in a variety of ward settings and provided a range of responses.

From the social survey it was found that the TNF indicator could differentiate ward sisters in terms of their therapeutic awareness. Areas of the indicator that were thought to be most sensitive in identifying the differences between ward sisters' attitudes were their definitions of the goal content, whether or not the sister carried out patient-centred care and their perceptions of the concept of rehabilitation. Possible limitations of the TNF indicator, however, rested with the fact that it was based on an ordinal scaling method and that its validity could be guaranteed only through acceptance of the theoretical framework. Despite these constraints, the indicator was able to distinguish patterns of behaviour and attitudes held by sisters who were aware of their therapeutic function and those who were less aware.

The relationship between ward sister's level of therapeutic awareness and the therapeutic content of self-care activities performed by and for patients was investigated by means of a case study in order to test the TNF indicator's validity in the ward setting. This more detailed case study of three ward environments not only demonstrated the accuracy of the TNF indicator as a predicitive scale for therapeutic and non-therapeutic ward sisters but also enabled other aspects of the theoretical framework to be developed more fully. The most important of these was the construction of a quality of care indicator, which graded self-care activities according to how effective they had been in achieving the goal of optimal self-care and independence for patients. This quality indicator was called the TNF matrix.

It was found that the therapeutic content of nursing activity was of a significantly higher standard in wards whose ward sister had a high TNF score than in wards where the sisters' TNF score was low. Variables such as improved ward environment or increased paramedical or medical involvement did not raise the therapeutic content of patients' self-care activities. The study also reflected the influence of the ward sister upon the approach that other members of the nursing staff took to their work. The findings showed that nurses who would have wanted to provide more patient-centred care were prevented from doing so where the ward sister had a low TNF score, whereas less therapeutically aware staff were able to provide better care in wards where the ward sisters had high TNF scores.

The main conclusion to be drawn from the findings was that the ward sister's concept of care, reflected in her TNF indicator score, was the most influential factor in determining the quality of patient care. Such a concept of care was seen as including a range of attributes and skills. Nurses who had this deeper understanding of their caring role demonstrated it in their problem-solving approach to individualised patient care. They saw the fundamental importance of assessing the individual self-care requirements of patients, of planning care and of identifying the range of assisting techniques that would be required to ensure that each patient was maintained at his optimal level of self-care. Included in the nurse's skill repertoire would be the ability to assess accurately patient mobility, functional ability and self-care potential. The nurse would also have to integrate individualised care of one patient with similar regimens for a ward of patients, a task requiring skill in organisation and management of resources. The nurse with a therapeutic approach to care would also be aware of her role in responding to patients' emotional and personal needs, ensuring dignity and self-worth in the face of physical and mental frailty. Quality of care could only be ensured when the concepts identified in relation to the nurse's therapeutic caring function were operationalised in the practice setting using the structure of the theoretical framework for geriatric nursing. Such a framework would ensure that nursing directs its activity on care and is not tempted by the medical goal or influenced by the custodial approach to care.

Thus, it was considered to be nursing's failure to identify the central importance of care and its failure to develop a theoretical framework capable of guiding and directing nursing action in the practice settings that was responsible for poor standards of patient care. Blame for the poor nursing standards could not be laid solely on the dominance of the geriatric medical model or on staffing and environmental constraints. The main problem was seen to lie with nursing's failure to define its therapeutic function in the care of the elderly. Despite the elucidating work of Norton et al (1962), nothing was done to construct a geriatric nursing model that would have given the necessary guidance and direction. Norton et al's recommendations to provide patient-centred care and to provide an environment that was therapeutic in meeting the needs of the elderly were not acted on. The knowledge and skills required for geriatric care were not identified within the profession, nor was any investment put into developing techniques of caring for the elderly hospitalised. Nursing practice seemed content to follow in the wake of medical innovation and change. In consequence, nursing was unable to consider seriously the complexities involved in providing care. Nursing also failed to look at the concept of care, failed to determine its essential components and failed to build a framework that would ensure the goal of care was achieved in the practice setting.

Nursing's caring role, or therapeutic function, can only be described within the overall structure of a theory that brings together those integral parts of nursing – the ability to identify patients' individual self-care needs, organise a system of care that is patient-dominated rather than task-oriented, identify the most appropriate nursing action to help to maintain a patient at his optimal level of self-care, and be able to provide a sensitive, personal and compassionate service that ensures patient dignity and self-respect. The TNF indicator was seen as an instrument that could be used to identify those characteristics in ward sisters, whereas the TNF matrix was a useful instrument with which to evaluate the quality of care. Both instruments were developed from the theoretical framework, which was based on the central premise of the importance of care; both instruments were seen as potentially useful indicators of the orientation and quality of geriatric nursing, not only to test the level of care but also to identify areas of improvement and to encourage nurses to develop their own knowledge and skills in order to provide even better care.

The final comment on the state of geriatric nursing is one of optimism, based on the belief that when nurses begin to accept and acknowledge *care* as the central most important concept in nursing, they will be able to define care in all its many dimensions, integrate it to a conceptual framework and use it in the practice setting. Caring will then be seen as involving not only the ability to organise, implement and manage but also the ability to act and do for, encourage, support, enthuse, counsel and comfort. This way, geriatric nursing will no longer be dominated by medical or other models, in that it will have developed its own conceptual framework with which to guide and direct care.

# Appendix I

THE TNF INDICATOR

---

**Section 1: Goal content**

1. How would you describe nursing in a geriatric ward? (What does geriatric nursing involve?)

2. Which of the following activities takes up most time on a geriatric ward? Please rank the activities listed below from 1 to 8, 1 for the activity that takes up most time, and 8 for that which takes up least of your time.

   a. Feeding patients, assisting patients with food
   b. Washing patients (not bathing)
   c. Caring for incontinent patients – washing, changing, cleaning
   d. Toiletting, commoding, toilet training
   e. Dressing/undressing patients
   f. Caring for pressure areas
   g. Exercising immobile patients
   h. Communicating with patients

3. Many nurses working with the elderly have described their work as involving the following activities. Please rank these activities in order of importance from 1 to 8, 1 for the activity that you think most important, and 8 for that which you consider least important.

   a. Carrying out medical treatment prescribed by the doctor
   b. Getting patients to move around and become more mobile
   c. Trying to teach and encourage patients to do things for themselves
   d. Keeping patients clean and comfortable
   e. Trying to create a relaxed atmosphere on the ward where patients feel 'at home'
   f. Caring for the physical needs of patients
   g. Stimulating patients to take an interest in surroundings and themselves
   h. Observing and recording medical progress of patients

222

## Section 2: Prescription/organisation and planning of nursing

### *Method of organising work on the ward*
1. What type of information do you make sure is collected from your patients to help assess and plan their nursing care?
2. How do you collect this information?
3. Who is responsible for collecting this information from the patients?
4. When this information is collected, where is it stored on the ward?
5. How do nurses working on the ward get access to this information?
6. What do you do with this information when it is collected?
7. Do you use structured nursing care plans to organise care for each patient on your ward?
8. When you have identified the nursing problems of your patients do you:

   a. inform your nursing staff and make a note of the problem(s) in the Kardex;
   b. list the problems and offer nursing measures to cope with them;
   c. make a written record of the problem(s) on the nursing care plan and offer nursing actions to solve them;
   d. carry on with the ward routine – most patient problems can be dealt with in the daily routine of care;
   e. carry on with the ward work observing for changes in the patient's condition and noting any change?

9. Do you usually set time limits within which you can expect problems to be solved?

   Always – noted in the nursing care plan
   Usually – written or expressed verbally
   Sometimes – keep a mental note of the situation
   Rarely – just don't know how things develop
   Never

10. How do you monitor the progress of your patients' conditions in relation to their nursing needs?
11. How do staff on the ward obtain information regarding the day-to-day progress and care of their patients?

    a. Daily nursing round with sister
    b. Direct involvement in the planning and organising of patient care by all grades of staff
    c. Reference to the nursing Kardex (individually reading and writing up reports and care given)

   d.  Reference to the nursing Kardex (collectively at report sessions
       in morning/afternoon/evening)
   e.  Informal communication of information between staff during
       work
   f.  Reference to patient progress charts attached to nursing care
       plans
   g.  Reference to information work-sheets

## Active management cycle

1. How do you inspect the daily needs of your patients? (Please tick.)

   a.  Gather up information from various sources about each
       patient as best you can
   b.  Make a point of seeing those patients who are ill and whose con-
       dition needs more careful consideration before delegating care
   c.  Check on/monitor patients' conditions while performing other
       jobs, e.g. medicine rounds, rounds with the Nursing Officer
       or medical rounds
   d.  Check on/monitor patients' progress while performing routine
       ward work with other members of staff
   e.  Make a point of going round each patient every
       morning/coming on duty and discussing their condition with
       them
   f.  Rely mainly on written reports and information from nursing
       staff during duty hours to monitor patients' needs

2. Which of the following methods of prescribing nursing work is
   closest to the system used on this ward?

   a.  There is a system of ward task lists in the form of procedure
       books, ward lists and duties for nurses
   b.  There is a set routine of work, which everyone knows about
   c.  There is a Kardex sheet for each patient on which instructions
       and comments are written by the ward sister and nurses
       caring for patients
   d.  There are individual work-sheets for each patient, updated by
       the ward sister each day, which set out details of care for the
       patient
   e.  There is a nursing care plan for each patient, setting out the
       details of care for the day

3. At the main report time of the day, when work is delegated to
   nurses, which of the following statements best describes the system
   of organising work on this ward?

a. A report is given by the ward sister to the trained staff on duty while the other nurses carry on with the routine ward work. After the report, the training staff, along with the other nurses start the routine work.

b. A report is given by the ward sister to all staff. Team leaders are appointed and delegated to care for a number of patients. Team leaders are responsible for the organisation of this work among their team members.

c. Ward sister and staff come together at the first opportunity and each patient's condition is discussed. The nursing workload is identified, and nurses themselves decide who will perform each task.

d. Ward sister and staff come together at a pre-arranged time (usually the morning) for a report. Each patient's nursing needs for the day are identified and each nurse is then given a plan of work to carry out for a group of patients.

e. No regular morning report is given by the ward sister. Most days, ward work follows the well-known routine of the ward.

4. There are *three* main ways of organising work on the ward. Which of the following items is closest to your own system?

a. Different nurses are organised to do just one particular job at a time for all patients on the ward

b. A group of nurses is allocated to one half of the ward and is reponsible for the care of all patients in that area of the ward

c. Nurses are given a group of patients to look after and do all the jobs for those patients

d. All three methods are used

e. Don't know

5. Here are some methods used by nurses in reporting back on their work to the ward sister. Please tick which is closest to your own system.

a. Ward sister receives verbal reports from all nurses on the morning shift on the work they have been responsible for carrying out

b. Ward sister receives verbal work reports from team leaders on the morning shift on the work their teams have carried out

c. Nurses write up nursing Kardex or sign work-lists when work is completed and only report to the ward sister on any important changes in patients

d. There is no organised system of reporting back on work in the ward

**Section 3: Survey list**

*Knowledge*

1. Do you feel that your general nursing training has prepared you adequately for the care of elderly patients?

   Yes          No          Don't know

2. Do qualified nurses working on a geriatric ward require special post-basic training to care for the elderly?

   Yes          No          Don't know

3. Do you feel there are any areas in geriatric nursing for which more education and training should be carried out?

   Yes          No          Don't know

   If yes, which areas?

*Skill utilisation*

1. Did you choose to come and work with the elderly on a geriatric ward?

   (Please tick one response.)

   a. Had no real choice, it was where they had a trained staff vacancy
   b. Had no choice at all
   c. Not really, it just happened that way
   d. Yes definitely, have always wanted to work with elderly people
   e. Yes, it was the most convenient job at the time
   f. Other reasons

2. In your present situation, do you feel that good use is being made of your skills? (Please tick.)

| **Skill** | **Utilisation** | | | | |
|---|---|---|---|---|---|
| | Very little use | Little use | Some use | Good use | Very good use |
| Basic nursing skills | ... | ... | ... | ... | ... |
| Rehabilitation skills | ... | ... | ... | ... | ... |

**Skill** **Utilisation**

| | Very little use | Little use | Some use | Good use | Very good use |
|---|---|---|---|---|---|
| Technical nursing skills | ... | ... | ... | ... | ... |
| Management skills | ... | ... | ... | ... | ... |
| Teaching skills | ... | ... | ... | ... | ... |
| Communication skills | ... | ... | ... | ... | ... |

3. Is there anything about your job that makes you really satisfied or gives you a feeling of accomplishment or achievement?

Yes          No

If yes, please tell me what it is.

## Concept of rehabilitation

1. How would you define the term 'rehabilitation'? (What does it involve?)
2. Please tell me what you consider to be the essential parts of an active rehabilitation programme of nursing care for:

   a. those patients on your ward who are termed 'rehabilitation patients';
   b. those patients who are termed 'long-stay/continuing care patients'.

3. What is the nurse's role in the rehabilitative care of her patients?

# Appendix II

## THE TNF INDICATOR SCALE

**Section 1: Goal content**

1. Definition of geriatric nursing (main features)

| TNF | 5 | 4 | 3 | 2 | 1 |
|-----|---|---|---|---|---|
| Response: | Maintenance/ rehabilitation therapy Total patient care | | Medical model orientation | | Routine care 'Just basic nursing care' |

2. Allocation of time according to nursing priorities

| TNF | 5 | 4 | 3 | 2 | 1 |
|-----|---|---|---|---|---|
| Response: | Toiletting Exercising Communicating | | Mix | | Others |

3. Ranking of activities

| TNF | 5 | 4 | 3 | 2 | 1 |
|-----|---|---|---|---|---|
| Response: | b, c, e, g | Mix | b, a, c, h | Mix | a, d, f, h |

# Section 2: Prescription/organisation and planning of nursing care

*Method of organising work on the ward*

**TNF**

| 3<br>*Problem-oriented care plan approach to nursing* | 2<br>*Semi-routinised approach* | 1<br>*Routinised approach to care* |
|---|---|---|
| 1. Reply includes: | | |
| a. Personal data – name, age, religion | a. Ditto | a. Ditto |
| b. Social data – occupation, dependents, housing | b. Ditto | b. Ditto |
| c. Health information – current diagnosis, present, past health problems, allergies | c. Ditto | c. Ditto |
| d. Patient's description of usual pattern of activities of daily living | d. Limited to diet, sleep, elimination | d. Diet, sleep, elimination |
| e. Emotional/psychological state<br>– from patient's point of view<br>– nurse's point of view | e. Data on emotional/psychological state of patient – as patient appears | |
| f. Patient's perception of cause of admission/health status | | |
| g. Comments of self-care ability and coping behaviour | | |
| 2. Nursing history/assessment sheet | Nursing history sheet/general format | Kardex/admission book/no predetermined format |
| | 1. Planned for needs of geriatric patients | |
| | 2. Adapted by ward sister for ward | |

**TNF 3**

| | 3 Problem-oriented care plan approach to nursing | 2 Semi-routinised approach | 1 Routinised approach to care |
|---|---|---|---|
| 3. | Delegate to any grade of nurse. Prerequisites: training in art of interviewing patient, use of nursing history form, ability to observe and perceive covert problems | Delegate to any grade of nurse. Use of loosely structured nursing history sheet/Kardex; little importance attached to interviewing | Delegate to junior nurses, auxiliaries. Routine admission procedure delegated to lowest nurse in ward; not seen as complex task |
| 4. | Stored with nursing care plans in filing systems | Kardex | Procedure books, admission books |
| 5. | Evidence of system whereby storage of information aids easy access, e.g. individual care plan folders + nursing history/information sheet – nurses free to consult patient care plans at any time or consult with team leader | Kardex system stored in sister's office. Information shared at regular report times or at request of staff; staff free to consult Kardex – may be prohibited by fact it is in sister's office | No organised system. Variety of books. Nurses are given information ad hoc or told to find out for themselves |
| 6. | After collecting information:<br>• Interpret it<br>• Define patient's nursing problems, i.e. establishing sources of possible problems and eliciting nursing intervention<br>• List priorities of care | • Plan nursing care – no evidence of problem-solving approach to nursing care | • Go on with routine care; information stored in Kardex, i.e. relevance of information in planning nursing care for individual patients not realised |
| 7. | Yes and reasons, e.g.:<br>• better method<br>• emphasises the individual care of the patient<br>• policy of health board<br>• efficient system<br>• helps students | It depends:<br>• Tried it but failed due to lack of staff<br>• Nursing care plan for ill patients | No<br>Not used because of:<br>• nursing shortage<br>• not liked<br>• plan to use<br>• task-oriented routine |

8. b. List the problems and offer nursing measures to cope with them
   c. Make a written record of the problem(s) on the nursing care plan and offer nursing actions to solve them
   a. Inform nursing staff and make a note of the problem(s) in the Kardex
   e. Carry on with the ward work observing for changes in the patient's condition and noting any change
   d. Carry on with the ward routine – most patient problems can be dealt with in the daily routine of care

9. Timing of goals legitimises 'evaluation procedure' – vital concept in problem-oriented approach
   Always – noted in the nursing care plan
   Usually – written or expressed verbally
   Sometimes – keep a mental note of the situation
   Slight evidence of awareness of need to time patients' reaction to nursing procedures
   Rarely – just don't know how things develop
   Never – not conceptually aware of the need for timing nursing; oriented to routine care; therefore, time is seen in terms of nurses getting work done rather than patients' progress

10. Monitor expected outcome with actual progress using parameters such as:
    - physiological/behavioural observations
    - patient's response to own situation
    - visual indications of progress
    - reassessment of problems

    Observation – general statement resting on physical and emotional state. Looking for comparative change based on experience and judgment rather than on planned nursing record
    - reassessment
    - medical round

    Observe – no explanation
    Nursing Kardex – no explanation
    Doctors' rounds – no explanation

11. Evidence of successful communication of instructions and progress:
    - specific instructions
    - giving both verbal and written instructions

    c. Reference to nursing Kardex individually
    d. Reference to nursing Kardex collectively at reports
    g. Reference to information work-sheets

    e. Information communication of information between staff during work
    d. Reference to nursing Kardex collectively at reports

| TNF 3 | 2 | 1 |
|---|---|---|
| *Problem-oriented care plan approach to nursing* | *Semi-routinised approach* | *Routinised approach to care* |
| a. Daily nursing rounds with sister | | |
| b. Direct involvement in the planning and organising of patient care by all grades of staff | | |
| f. Reference to patient progress charts attached to nursing care plans | | |

## Active management cycle

| TNF 3 | 2 | 1 |
|---|---|---|
| *Complete* | *Incomplete* | *Not performed* |

1. Nursing round of patients

| TNF 3 | 2 | 1 |
|---|---|---|
| e. Make a point of going round each patient every morning/on coming on duty and discussing their condition with them | b. Make a point of seeing those patients who are ill and whose condition needs more careful consideration before delegating care | d. Check on/monitor patients' progress while performing routine ward work with other members of staff |
| | c. Check on/monitor patients' condition while performing other jobs, e.g. medicine rounds, rounds with the Nursing Officer or medical rounds | f. Rely mainly on written reports and information from nursing staff during duty hours to monitor patients' needs |
| | | a. Gather up information from various sources about each patient as best as one can |

2. Written work prescription – criterion: evidence of daily prospective work prescription for each patient

   a. There is a system of ward task lists in the form of procedure books, ward lists and duties for nurses

   b. There is a set routine of work, which everyone knows about

   c. There is a Kardex sheet for each patient on which instructions and comments are written by the ward sister and nurses caring for patients

   d. There are individual work-sheets for each patient, updated by the ward sister each day, which set out details of care for the patient

   e. There is a nursing care plan for each patient, setting out details of care for the day

3. Verbal work prescription – criteria: (1) planned time near beginning of shift when all nurses receive work prescription for the day; (2) evidence of each patient having been identified in relation to work prescription; (3) evidence of each nurse being allocated work

   a. A report is given by the ward sister to trained staff on duty while the other nurses carry on with the routine ward work. After report trained staff, along with other nurses, start the routine work

   b. A report is given by the ward sister to all staff. Team leaders are appointed and delegated to care for a number of patients. Team leaders are responsible for the organisation of this work among their team members

   c. Ward sister and staff come together at the first opportunity and each patient's condition is discussed. The nursing workload is identified and nurses themselves decide who will perform each task

   d. Ward sister and staff come together at a pre-arranged time (usually the morning) for a report. Each patient's nursing needs for the day are identified and each nurse is then given a plan of work to carry out for a group of patients

   e. No regular morning report is given by the ward sister. Most days, ward work follows the well-known routine of the ward

4. Allocation:

   a. Different nurses are organised to do just one particular job at a time for all patients on the ward

      (ward allocation/task-oriented)

   b. A group of nurses is allocated to one half of the ward and are responsible for the care of all patients in that area of the ward

      (geographical allocation, groups of nurses and groups of patients)

   c. Nurses are given a group of patients to look after and do all the jobs for those patients

      (patient allocation, multi-skilled, individual responsibility)

   d. There is no organised system of reporting back on work in the ward

5. Accountability:

   a. Ward sister receives verbal reports from all nurses on the morning shift on the work they have been responsible for carrying out

   b. Ward sister receives verbal report from team leader on the morning shift on the work their teams have carried out

   c. Nurses write up nursing Kardex or sign work-lists when work is completed and only report to the ward sister on any important changes in patients

# Section 3: Survey list
## Knowledge
### TNF 3

1. Feeling that general training has not prepared one adequately for care of elderly

   1 Satisfied with general training

2. Agree: nurses need special post-basic training courses

   2 Disagree: nurses do not need special training

3. Identified more than three areas in which more education and training were required, e.g. rehabilitation, psychological aspects of care, process of ageing, multiple pathologies, diversional therapy

   Felt no extra training was needed

## Skill utilisation

### 1. Choice of ward

**TNF**

| 3 | 2 | 1 |
|---|---|---|
| Yes definitely, have always wanted to work with elderly people | | No, had no choice at all |

### 2. Skill

**TNF**

| 5 | 4 | 3 | 2 | 1 |
|---|---|---|---|---|
| Very good use | Good use | Some use | Little use | Very little use |

For:
Basic nursing skills
Rehabilitation skills
Technical nursing skills
Management skills
Teaching skills
Communication skills

### 3. Job satisfaction

**TNF**

| 5 | 4 | 3 | 2 | 1 |
|---|---|---|---|---|
| Total patient care approach | Rehabilitation | Medical model goals | Personal | Basic/routine nursing care goals |

*Concept of rehabilitation*

| TNF | 5 | 4 | 3 | 2 | 1 |
|---|---|---|---|---|---|
| | | *Therapeutic* | | *Non-therapeutic* | |
| 1. Definition of rehabilitation | | • To restore patient to maximum potential<br>• To ensure patient is given correct aids and equipment<br>• Involves gradual reduction in amount of aid/supervision given by staff as patient gains confidence | | Lack of awareness of these features | |
| 2a. Essential parts of active rehabilitation programme for rehabilitation patients | | • Time<br>• Mental assessment<br>• Realistic goal setting<br>• Stimulation of desire for self-help | | Lack of awareness of these features | |
| 2b. Essential parts of active rehabilitation programme for continuing care patients | | • Maintenance therapy<br>• Diversional therapy<br>• Emphasis on prevention of deterioration | | Lack of awareness of these features | |
| 3. Definition of nursing role in rehabilitation of patients | | • To know individual potential of each patient<br>• To give proper nursing assistance<br>• To strive to provide an environment therapeutic to each individual and to enhance improvement | | Lack of awareness of these features | |

# Appendix III

## TNF INDICATOR RESULTS

| TNF indicator scores | | | Maximum possible score | White Ward | Brown Ward | Red Ward |
|---|---|---|:---:|:---:|:---:|:---:|
| **Section 1** | 1. | Definition of geriatric nursing | 5 | 5 | 3 | 2 |
| Goal | 2. | Ranking activities | 5 | 5 | 2 | 2 |
| content | 3. | Time spent | 5 | 4 | 1 | 3 |
| **Section 2** | a. | Type of information collected | 3 | 3 | 2 | 1 |
| Prescription | b. | Method of data collection | 3 | 3 | 2 | 2 |
| of individual | c. | Method of communication | 3 | 2 | 1 | 1 |
| patient | d. | Information storage | 3 | 2 | 2 | 2 |
| care | e. | Access to nursing staff | 3 | 3 | 2 | 2 |
| | f. | Use of information | 3 | 3 | 1 | 1 |
| | g. | Problem identification | 3 | 3 | 2 | 2 |
| | h. | Setting time limits | 3 | 2 | 1 | 1 |
| | i. | Monitoring patient progress | 3 | 2 | 2 | 2 |
| | j. | Informing staff | 3 | 3 | 1 | 2 |
| | k. | Obtaining information | 3 | 2 | 1 | 2 |
| Active | a. | Monitoring daily needs | 3 | 3 | 1 | 1 |
| management | b. | Method of work presentation | 3 | 2 | 2 | 2 |
| cycle | c. | Work delegation | 3 | 3 | 2 | 1 |
| | d. | Method of work organisation | 3 | 3 | 1 | 1 |
| | e. | Work accountability | 3 | 3 | 2 | 2 |
| Survey | 1. | Nurse training | 3 | 3 | 1 | 1 |
| list | 2. | Post-basic training | 3 | 3 | 2 | 3 |
| | 3. | Specialist areas | 3 | 3 | 2 | 2 |
| Skill | A. | Ward choice | 3 | 3 | 3 | 2 |
| utilisation | | 1. Basic skills | 5 | 5 | 4 | 4 |
| | | 2. Rehabilitation | 5 | 5 | 5 | 4 |
| | | 3. Technical | 5 | 5 | 4 | 4 |
| | | 4. Managerial | 5 | 5 | 4 | 4 |
| | | 5. Teaching | 5 | 5 | 5 | 4 |
| | | 6. Communicating | 5 | 5 | 5 | 4 |
| | B. | Satisfaction with work | 5 | 5 | 2 | 2 |
| Rehabilitation | 1. | Definition | 5 | 5 | 3 | 3 |
| concept | 2. | Active rehabilitation | 5 | 5 | 4 | 3 |
| | 3. | Active rehabilitation for continuing care patients | 5 | 5 | 4 | 2 |
| | 4. | Nurse's role | 5 | 5 | 4 | 2 |
| *Total* | | | 130 | 123 | 83 | 76 |

# Appendix IV

OBSERVATION SCHEDULE

| Time (a.m.) | 1 W/C | 2 S/E | 3 W/C | 4 P/C | 5 W/C | 6 P/C | 7 S/E | 8 S/E |
|---|---|---|---|---|---|---|---|---|
| | | | | | Ward | | | |
| 8.00 | Bed | Up at bedside getting dress on | Sitting at bedside eating porridge | Sitting at bedside eating bread | Bed | Asked what he wants for breakfast – porridge. | Bed | Bed |
| 8.06 | Bed | At bedside. Nurse tying shoes | At bedside looking for clips in drawer | At bedside eating bread | Fed porridge by N/A, given tea in feeding cup. Patient is very low in bed – left to drink tea like this | Radio on, putting teeth in. Bed table pushed through cot sides: awkward for patient – difficulty in eating porridge | Given breakfast. Cot sides remain up | Cup set out for patient. Porridge in a plate |
| 8.12 | Bed | At bedside putting on cardigan | At bedside looking for clips | Bedside, quiet | Still quite far down bed – attempting to drink tea | Eating bread on lap in bed | Eating bread. Cotsides still up | N/A feeding patient porridge |

**Ward**

| Time (a.m.) | 1 W/C | 2 S/E | 3 W/C | 4 P/C | 5 W/C | 6 P/C | 7 S/E | 8 S/E |
|---|---|---|---|---|---|---|---|---|
| 8.18 | Bed | Washing hands at sink, standing with Zimmer frame, combing hair | N/A asking patient if she needs a wash 'underneath', asking her if she needs a clean Kanga pad. Sorting out laundry | Nightie off, looking for something in bed | Drinking tea with difficulty, eating bread | Drinking tea in bed | Using urinal, drinking tea | Being fed by N/A; given tea. Patient left with some bread and tea. Was able to eat bread but unable to tip cup far enough back to get fluid. Comment from nurse: 'You're doing to spill that tea!' |
| 8.24 | Bed | In day-room looking in bag | N/A helping patient with clothes – vest and slip. Patient asking for a lighter cardigan | Sitting motionless at bedside with just vest on | Still drinking tea | Sitting in bed, cotsides up | In bed, smoking. No attempt to get patient started to dress self. No curtains round bed | Tea cup taken from patient. No alternative. |

| Time (a.m.) | 1 W/C | 2 S/E | 3 W/C | 4 P/C | 5 W/C | 6 P/C | 7 S/E | 8 S/E |
|---|---|---|---|---|---|---|---|---|
| | | | | | Ward | | | |
| 8.30 | Bed | Sitting in day-room looking round | Two nurses setting patient on sanichair | Sitting motionless at bedside, still in same state | In bed. Nurse in with patient telling him to roll over and grab bar. Telling him to roll back | Nurse in with patient dressing him | Nurse asking patient if he had a good day out at weekend. Nurse took pyjama top off, dressing patient without getting him to help her. | Bed |
| 8.36 | Bed | Sitting in day-room | Wheeled up to toilet | Dressed by N/A. No attempt to get patient to help in process. Wheeled over to toilet and asked to wait | Trousers put on by nurse. Little comment | Being dressed by nurse. No attempt to get patient to help | Being completely dressed by nurse | Bed |
| 8.42 | Bed | Sitting in day-room looking round | Sitting on toilet, door left open – patient exposed to corridor | In toilet, door ajar | At bedside, upper half being dressed | Sitting on sanichair being dressed by N/A; given tablet. Radio turned over to another channel by nurse – not at request of | Nurse continuing to dress patient completely | Bed |

Ward

| Time (a.m.) | 1 W/C | 2 S/E | 3 W/C | 4 P/C | 5 W/C | 6 P/C | 7 S/E | 8 S/E |
|---|---|---|---|---|---|---|---|---|
| 8.48 | Bed | Sitting in day-room, quiet | On toilet calling 'I'm ready' | Taken off sanichair. Stood up (first time) and walked over to physio-therapy. Rather unsteady on feet. Stockings falling down | Given flannel to wash hands and face. Told to do this by nurse | Wheeled out to toilet on sanichair | Sitting in seat beside bed. Told nurse he had washed himself(!) | Bed |
| 8.54 | Bed | Sitting in day-room, quiet | On toilet calling for nurse | Physiotherapy | Sitting by window in ward bay in wheelchair | In toilet, door ajar | Sitting in chair smoking | Being got out of bed by nurse. Underpants being put on. No communication between patient and nurse |

*Key:* W/C – Wholly compensatory
P/C – Partly compensatory
S/E – Supportive – educative

**White Ward**

| Time (a.m.) | 1 W/C | 2 S/E | 3 W/C | 4 P/C | 5 W/C | 6 P/C | 7 S/E | 8 S/E |
|---|---|---|---|---|---|---|---|---|
| 8.00 | Curtains round bed, sanichair in. Nurse working with patient | Sitting up in bed | Curtains round patient sitting in bed | Nurse in with patient getting her ready to go to toilet | Curtains round patient putting on stockings and bra. Nurse gone to get sanichair for patient | Curtains round dressing self | Bed | Bed |
| 8.06 | On sanichair being wheeled up to toilet | In bed, sitting | Nurse in with patient helping her to put stockings on | On sanichair | Wheeled back from toilet | Walked out to toilet with Zimmer aid. Staff nurse wheeled sanichair into toilet | Bed | Bed |
| 8.12 | Toilet | Bed | Sitting on sanichair at bedside | On sanichair calling for nurse | Sitting on chair dressing self | Walked back to bed. Washing self there | Bed | Bed |
| 8.18 | Wheeled back from toilet by N/A | Bed, Sdt/N giving patient medicine – Sister showing her better way of doing it | Patient wheeled to toilet on sanichair | S/N dressing patient – explaining what she's doing as she goes on | Dressing self behind curtain | Dressing/ washing self | Bed | Bed |

| Time | | | | | | | | |
|------|---|---|---|---|---|---|---|---|
| 8.24 | Sitting in Buxton chair at bedside, basin in front, hairbrush in hand | Sitting in bed; taking teeth out. Nurse asking if she has finished her medicine | Basin in front of her; sitting on easy chair with cantilever table | S/N with patient helping her to wash face and hands | Sitting on chair at bedside | Curtains round still washing self | Bed | Bed |
| 8.30 | Folding/rolling bandages with hand | N/A washing patient's bottom behind curtains | Sitting on chair drinking dorbinex | Sitting at bedside dressed | Sitting at bedside dressed | Dressing | Bed | Bed |
| 8.36 | Still rolling bandages | Two nurses in with patient washing and dressing her | Sitting on chair in ward bay | Sitting quietly | Sitting looking at a book | Still organising self | Bed | Bed |
| 8.42 | Sitting quietly | N/A wheeling patient out to toilet | Sitting | Sitting | Sitting | Still organising self | Bed | Bed |
| 8.48 | Sitting in chair, breakfast served. Eating porridge by self – given non-slip mat for plate – able to manage despite paralysed right arm | Back from toilet; transferred from sanichair to Buxton chair by two nurses – standing patient up at bars in corridor, pulling knickers up and setting her on Buxton chair | Sitting quietly | Sitting | Sitting | Organising self | Bed | N/A in with patient telling her she is going to wash patient's bottom and put dry clothes on |

**White Ward**

| Time (a.m.) | 1 W/C | 2 S/E | 3 W/C | 4 P/C | 5 W/C | 6 P/C | 7 S/E | 8 S/E |
|---|---|---|---|---|---|---|---|---|
| 8.54 | Eating breakfast – independent and managing well | N/A, after washing patient's teeth, told her to put them in herself. Patient put them in soapy water in front of her. N/A patiently explaining how to put teeth in her mouth | Sitting quietly | S/N giving out serviettes to patient; asked if she would like cereal – requested porridge | Asked for cornflakes, eating breakfast | Choice of cereal – eating breakfast | Bed | At bedside. N/A asking for help to transfer patient from bedside to Buxton chair. Good transfer |

*Key:*  W/C – Wholly compensatory
P/C – Partly compensatory
S/E – Supportive – educative

# Appendix V

## CODING LIST

---

01 Elimination
02 Feeding
03 Washing
04 Bathing
05 Dressing
06 Undressing
07 Exercising
08 Communicating
09 Medicines
10 Drinking
11 Day-room (engaged)
12 Day-room (passive)
13 In bed
14 Sitting in a chair at bedside/in ward bay (engaged)
15 Sitting in a chair at bedside/in ward bay (passive)
16 Sitting at bedside (engaged)
17 Sitting at bedside (passive)
18 Weighed
19 Visitors
20 Physiotherapy (engaged)
21 Physiotherapy (passive)
22 Occupational therapy (engaged)
23 Occupational therapy (passive)
24 Doctor visiting/medical round
25 Chiropodist
26 Art therapy
27 Minister of religion
28 Hairdresser/barber
29 Social worker
30 Lifted out of bed
31 Put into bed
32 Lifting out of chair
33 Transfer from physiotherapy to ward or vice versa, by porter
34 Patient distressed
35 Patient out with relatives
36 Dressings
37 Smoking

# Appendix VI

## CODING FRAME

| Label | Code | | | | |
|---|---|---|---|---|---|
| SERN | 0 | 9 | | | |
| CDN | 1 | 1 | | | |
| WDN | 2 | | | | |
| DPA | 0 | 2 | | | |
| DPB | 0 | 3 | | | |
| AGE | 8 | 4 | | | |
| SEX | 2 | | | | |
| TYPT | 1 | | | | |
| TIME | 1 | | | | |
| DAY | 1 | | | | |
| A1 | 1 | 3 | 0 | 0 | 0 |
| 2 | 0 | 5 | 3 | 2 | 2 |
| 3 | 0 | 1 | 2 | 2 | 2 |
| 4 | 0 | 1 | 2 | 2 | 2 |
| 5 | 0 | 3 | 2 | 2 | 2 |
| 6 | 0 | 3 | 2 | 2 | 2 |
| 7 | 1 | 5 | 0 | 0 | 0 |
| 8 | 1 | 5 | 0 | 0 | 0 |
| 9 | 0 | 2 | 2 | 2 | 2 |
| 10 | 0 | 2 | 2 | 2 | 2 |
| 11 | 1 | 4 | 0 | 0 | 0 |
| 12 | 1 | 4 | 0 | 0 | 0 |
| 13 | 1 | 2 | 0 | 0 | 0 |
| SERN | 0 | 9 | | | |
| CDN | 2 | 2 | | | |
| DAY | 1 | | | | |
| 14 | 1 | 2 | 0 | 0 | 0 |
| 15 | 1 | 2 | 0 | 0 | 0 |
| 16 | 1 | 2 | 0 | 0 | 0 |
| 17 | 1 | 2 | 0 | 0 | 0 |
| 18 | 1 | 2 | 0 | 0 | 0 |
| 19 | 1 | 2 | 0 | 0 | 0 |
| 20 | 1 | 2 | 0 | 0 | 0 |
| 21 | 1 | 2 | 0 | 0 | 0 |
| 22 | 1 | 2 | 0 | 0 | 0 |
| 23 | 1 | 2 | 0 | 0 | 0 |
| 24 | 1 | 2 | 0 | 0 | 0 |
| 25 | 1 | 2 | 0 | 0 | 0 |
| 26 | 1 | 2 | 0 | 0 | 0 |
| 27 | 1 | 0 | 0 | 0 | 1 |
| 28 | 1 | 2 | 0 | 0 | 0 |
| SERN | 0 | 9 | | | |
| CDN | 1 | 3 | | | |
| DAY | 1 | | | | |
| 29 | 1 | 2 | 0 | 0 | 0 |
| 30 | 1 | 2 | 0 | 0 | 0 |
| 31 | 1 | 2 | 0 | 0 | 0 |
| 32 | 1 | 2 | 0 | 0 | 0 |
| 33 | 1 | 2 | 0 | 0 | 0 |
| 34 | 1 | 2 | 0 | 0 | 0 |
| 35 | 1 | 2 | 0 | 0 | 0 |
| 36 | 1 | 2 | 0 | 0 | 0 |
| 37 | 1 | 2 | 0 | 0 | 0 |
| 38 | 1 | 2 | 0 | 0 | 0 |
| 39 | 1 | 2 | 0 | 0 | 0 |
| 40 | 0 | 2 | 2 | 2 | 2 |
| ST | 0 | 7 | | | |
| NUR | 0 | 1 | 0 | 2 | 4 |

| Label | Code | | | | |
|---|---|---|---|---|---|
| SERN | 0 | 9 | | | |
| CDN | 2 | 1 | | | |
| WDN | 2 | | | | |
| DPA | 0 | 2 | | | |
| DPB | 0 | 3 | | | |
| AGE | 8 | 4 | | | |
| SEX | 2 | | | | |
| TYPT | 1 | | | | |
| TIME | 2 | | | | |
| DAY | 1 | | | | |
| A1 | 1 | 2 | 2 | 2 | 2 |
| 2 | 0 | 2 | 2 | 2 | 2 |
| 3 | 0 | 2 | 2 | 2 | 2 |
| 4 | 1 | 2 | 0 | 0 | 0 |
| 5 | 1 | 2 | 0 | 0 | 0 |
| 6 | 1 | 2 | 0 | 0 | 0 |
| 7 | 0 | 1 | 2 | 2 | 2 |
| 8 | 0 | 1 | 2 | 2 | 2 |
| 9 | 0 | 1 | 2 | 2 | 2 |
| 10 | 1 | 2 | 0 | 0 | 0 |
| 11 | 1 | 2 | 0 | 0 | 0 |
| 12 | 1 | 2 | 0 | 0 | 0 |
| 13 | 1 | 2 | 0 | 0 | 0 |
| SERN | 0 | 9 | | | |
| CDN | 2 | 2 | | | |
| DAY | 2 | | | | |
| 14 | 1 | 2 | 0 | 0 | 0 |
| 15 | 1 | 2 | 0 | 0 | 0 |
| 16 | 1 | 0 | 0 | 0 | 1 |
| 17 | 1 | 2 | 0 | 0 | 0 |
| 18 | 1 | 2 | 0 | 0 | 0 |
| 19 | 1 | 2 | 0 | 0 | 0 |
| 20 | 0 | 8 | 3 | 2 | 2 |
| 21 | 1 | 2 | 0 | 0 | 0 |
| 22 | 1 | 2 | 0 | 0 | 0 |
| 23 | 0 | 7 | 3 | 2 | 2 |
| 24 | 0 | 7 | 3 | 2 | 2 |
| 25 | 1 | 9 | 0 | 0 | 1 |
| 26 | 1 | 1 | 0 | 0 | 1 |
| 27 | 1 | 2 | 0 | 0 | 0 |
| 28 | 1 | 2 | 0 | 0 | 0 |
| SERN | 0 | 9 | | | |
| CDN | 2 | 3 | | | |
| DAY | 1 | | | | |
| 29 | 1 | 2 | 0 | 0 | 0 |
| 30 | 1 | 2 | 0 | 0 | 0 |
| 31 | 1 | 2 | 0 | 0 | 0 |
| 32 | 1 | 2 | 0 | 0 | 0 |
| 33 | 1 | 2 | 0 | 0 | 0 |
| 34 | 1 | 2 | 0 | 0 | 0 |
| 35 | 1 | 2 | 0 | 0 | 0 |
| 36 | 1 | 2 | 0 | 0 | 0 |
| 37 | 0 | 1 | 2 | 2 | 2 |
| 38 | 0 | 1 | 2 | 2 | 2 |
| 39 | 1 | 2 | 0 | 0 | 0 |
| 40 | 1 | 2 | 0 | 0 | 0 |
| ST | 0 | 7 | | | |
| NUR | 1 | 0 | 1 | 3 | 2 |

| Label | Code | | | | |
|---|---|---|---|---|---|
| SERN | 0 | 9 | | | |
| CDN | 3 | 1 | | | |
| WDN | 2 | | | | |
| DPA | 0 | 2 | | | |
| DPB | 0 | 3 | | | |
| AGE | 8 | 4 | | | |
| SEX | 2 | | | | |
| TYPT | 1 | | | | |
| TIME | 3 | | | | |
| DAY | 1 | | | | |
| A1 | 1 | 2 | 0 | 0 | 0 |
| 2 | 1 | 2 | 0 | 0 | 0 |
| 3 | 0 | 1 | 2 | 2 | 2 |
| 4 | 0 | 1 | 2 | 2 | 2 |
| 5 | 0 | 1 | 2 | 2 | 2 |
| 6 | 1 | 1 | 0 | 0 | 0 |
| 7 | 1 | 1 | 0 | 0 | 0 |
| 8 | 0 | 8 | 3 | 2 | 2 |
| 9 | 0 | 2 | 2 | 2 | 2 |
| 10 | 0 | 2 | 2 | 2 | 2 |
| 11 | 0 | 2 | 2 | 2 | 2 |
| 12 | 1 | 2 | 0 | 0 | 0 |
| 13 | 1 | 2 | 0 | 0 | 0 |
| SERN | 0 | 9 | | | |
| CDN | 3 | 2 | | | |
| DAY | 1 | | | | |
| 14 | 1 | 2 | 0 | 0 | 0 |
| 15 | 0 | 1 | 2 | 2 | 2 |
| 16 | 0 | 1 | 2 | 2 | 2 |
| 17 | 0 | 6 | 2 | 2 | 3 |
| 18 | 0 | 3 | 2 | 2 | 3 |
| 19 | 0 | 8 | 3 | 2 | 2 |
| 20 | 1 | 3 | 0 | 0 | 0 |
| 21 | 1 | 3 | 0 | 0 | 0 |
| 22 | 1 | 3 | 0 | 0 | 0 |
| 23 | 1 | 3 | 0 | 0 | 0 |
| 24 | 1 | 3 | 0 | 0 | 0 |
| 25 | 1 | 3 | 0 | 0 | 0 |
| 26 | 1 | 3 | 0 | 0 | 0 |
| 27 | 1 | 3 | 0 | 0 | 0 |
| 28 | 1 | 3 | 0 | 0 | 0 |
| SERN | 0 | 9 | | | |
| CDN | 3 | 3 | | | |
| DAY | 1 | | | | |
| 29 | 1 | 3 | 0 | 0 | 0 |
| 30 | 1 | 3 | 0 | 0 | 0 |
| 31 | 1 | 3 | 0 | 0 | 0 |
| 32 | 1 | 3 | 0 | 0 | 0 |
| 33 | 1 | 3 | 0 | 0 | 0 |
| 34 | 1 | 3 | 0 | 0 | 0 |
| 35 | 1 | 3 | 0 | 0 | 0 |
| 36 | 1 | 3 | 0 | 0 | 0 |
| 37 | 1 | 3 | 0 | 0 | 0 |
| 38 | 1 | 3 | 0 | 0 | 0 |
| 39 | 1 | 3 | 0 | 0 | 0 |
| 40 | 1 | 3 | 0 | 0 | 0 |
| ST | 0 | 4 | | | |
| NUR | 1 | 0 | 0 | 1 | 2 |

# Appendix VII

## TNF MATRIX

| Level of therapeutic activity | Nursing system | Initiation | Process | Outcome | |
|---|---|---|---|---|---|
| Optimally therapeutic action | Supportive – educative | Patient-initiated and facilitated, nurse-for patient-initiated and positively facilitated | Functional ability Mobility facility | Optimal utilisation – independent; nurse supervision | *Success* independence |
| 4 | Partly compensatory | Patient-initiated, nurse positive facilitated | Functional ability Mobility facility | Optimal utilisation; nurse supported | *Success* nursing help |
| | Wholly compensatory | Nurse-for-patient initiated and facilitated | Functional ability Mobility facility | Optimal utilisation Nurse assistance | *Success* nurse-directed and controlled; appropriate action |
| Moderately therapeutic action | Supportive – educative | Nurse-initiated, patient-limited facilitation; patient-initiated, limited facilitation | Functional ability Mobility facility | Limited utilisation | *Limited success* below optimum independence |
| 3 | Partly compensatory | Patient-initiated, nurse-limited facilitation | Functional ability Mobility facility | Limited utilisation | *Limited success* limited help/supervision |
| | Wholly compensatory | Nurse-for-patient initiated, limited facilitation | Functional ability Mobility facility | Limited utilisation | *Limited success* limited nurse direction/control-/action |
| Minimally therapeutic action | Supportive – educative | Nurse-initiated, minimal patient facilitation | Functional ability Mobility facility | Minimal utilisation | *Minimal success* minimal independence |
| 2 | Partly compensatory | Nurse-initiated, minimal patient facilitation | Functional ability Mobility facility | Minimal utilisation | *Minimal success* minimal help/supervision |
| | Wholly compensatory | Nurse-without-patient initiated, minimal facilitation | Functional ability Mobility facility | Minimal utilisation | *Minimal success* inappropriate nurse direction/control /action |

| Level of therapeutic activity | Nursing system | Initiation | Process | Outcome | |
|---|---|---|---|---|---|
| Non-therapeutic action | Supportive – educative | Nurse-without-patient initiated; inadequate facilitation | Functional ability Mobility facility | Inadequate utilisation | *Unsuccessful* loss of independence |
| 1 | Partly compensatory | Nurse-without-patient initiated; inadequate facilitation | Functional ability Mobility facility | Inadequate utilisation | *Unsuccessful* inadequate help/supervision |
| | Wholly compensatory | Nurse-without-patient initiated; inadequate facilitation | Functional ability Mobility facility | Inadequate utilisation | *Unsuccessful* inadequate nurse direction/control of action |

# Appendix VIII

PERCENTAGE TIME SPENT IN CERTAIN ACTIVITIES
BY GERIATRIC PATIENTS IN THREE WARDS

| | Brown Ward –TNF | | | | | | | | White Ward +TNF | | | | | | | | Red Ward –TNF | | | | | | | |
|---|---|---|---|---|---|---|---|---|---|---|---|---|---|---|---|---|---|---|---|---|---|---|---|---|
| Patient: | 1 | 2 | 3 | 4 | 5 | 6 | 7 | 8 | 1 | 2 | 3 | 4 | 5 | 6 | 7 | 8 | 1 | 2 | 3 | 4 | 5 | 6 | 7 | 8 |
| Nursing system: | W/C | W/C | W/C | P/C | P/C | S/E | S/E | S/E | W/C | W/C | W/C | P/C | P/C | P/C | P/C | S/E | W/C | W/C | W/C | P/C | P/C | P/C | P/C | S/E |
| **Self-care activities** | | | | | | | | | | | | | | | | | | | | | | | | |
| Elimination | 0.4 | 5.1 | 3.1 | 5.0 | 6.3 | 1.9 | 2.3 | 2.5 | 1.5 | 4.5 | 7.0 | 4.8 | 4.0 | 4.0 | 8.2 | 2.5 | 1.2 | 1.9 | 4.8 | 3.0 | 4.6 | 3.1 | 1.1 | 4.4 |
| Feeding | 6.7 | 5.8 | 11.2 | 8.2 | 6.3 | 9.0 | 10.4 | 7.0 | 9.6 | 9.0 | 7.9 | 8.1 | 6.9 | 9.6 | 6.5 | 8.0 | 7.5 | 5.7 | 6.3 | 5.0 | 8.6 | 6.5 | 5.2 | 7.4 |
| Drinking | 1.0 | 3.5 | 3.0 | 3.2 | 2.1 | 3.0 | 2.3 | 3.2 | 2.3 | 2.3 | 2.3 | 3.2 | 2.0 | 4.2 | 2.5 | 1.9 | 4.8 | 0.0 | 1.8 | 2.3 | 2.9 | 2.0 | 1.0 | 1.8 |
| Washing | 2.9 | 1.1 | 2.3 | 1.8 | 1.2 | 0.2 | 2.5 | 0.5 | 2.3 | 2.4 | 1.9 | 1.1 | 0.7 | 2.4 | 1.4 | 2.5 | 2.6 | 2.4 | 1.1 | 1.1 | 1.8 | 0.7 | 2.0 | 3.0 |
| Bathing | 0.0 | 0.0 | 0.2 | 0.1 | 0.1 | 0.4 | 1.1 | 0.4 | 0.5 | 0.1 | 0.0 | 0.0 | 0.7 | 0.8 | 0.4 | 0.2 | 0.6 | 0.0 | 0.0 | 0.5 | 0.6 | 0.0 | 0.0 | 0.1 |
| Dressing | 1.4 | 1.4 | 0.6 | 1.9 | 1.3 | 2.7 | 0.8 | 2.0 | 0.5 | 1.3 | 0.8 | 1.0 | 1.2 | 0.8 | 1.7 | 3.8 | 0.8 | 1.3 | 1.0 | 1.1 | 1.9 | 1.0 | 1.7 | 3.9 |
| Undressing | 0.8 | 1.3 | 1.2 | 1.3 | 1.0 | 0.5 | 0.6 | 2.3 | 1.3 | 1.3 | 1.3 | 0.4 | 1.8 | 0.7 | 1.9 | 2.3 | 0.8 | 1.8 | 0.0 | 1.7 | 1.3 | 1.4 | 1.0 | 2.0 |
| Exercising | 0.0 | 0.0 | 0.0 | 0.8 | 3.6 | 4.0 | 1.5 | 3.6 | 0.0 | 0.6 | 0.7 | 0.1 | 5.0 | 2.9 | 0.5 | 4.3 | 0.0 | 0.0 | 0.0 | 1.7 | 6.8 | 7.0 | 8.5 | 8.0 |
| Communication | 0.5 | 1.2 | 2.4 | 4.2 | 1.5 | 1.4 | 0.8 | 1.9 | 2.7 | 2.4 | 1.5 | 4.2 | 6.0 | 2.3 | 1.9 | 3.0 | 2.0 | 1.5 | 2.7 | 3.5 | 0.6 | 1.3 | 5.2 | 1.8 |
| **Contact** | | | | | | | | | | | | | | | | | | | | | | | | |
| Doctor | 0.0 | 0.0 | 0.0 | 0.5 | 0.1 | 0.0 | 0.4 | 0.2 | 0.2 | 0.0 | 0.0 | 0.0 | 0.0 | 0.0 | 0.1 | 0.1 | 0.0 | 0.0 | 0.0 | 0.1 | 0.2 | 0.2 | 0.0 | 0.0 |
| Physiotherapist | 0.0 | 0.0 | 0.0 | 4.8 | 0.0 | 0.0 | 4.7 | 8.3 | 0.0 | 3.8 | 0.0 | 0.0 | 5.1 | 0.0 | 2.4 | 5.0 | 11.9 | 1.0 | 2.8 | 0.0 | 4.6 | 0.0 | 5.3 | 7.5 |
| Occupational therapist | 0.0 | 0.0 | 0.0 | 0.0 | 8.8 | 0.0 | 0.6 | 0.0 | 0.0 | 0.0 | 0.0 | 0.0 | 1.0 | 0.0 | 0.7 | 0.0 | 12.0 | 0.0 | 1.6 | 0.0 | 3.9 | 0.0 | 1.4 | 8.1 |
| Others | 0.0 | 0.0 | 0.7 | 0.8 | 1.8 | 0.0 | 0.7 | 0.8 | 0.0 | 1.4 | 0.0 | 0.0 | 0.4 | 0.6 | 2.7 | 0.2 | 1.0 | 33.5 | 0.0 | 1.0 | 0.1 | 0.0 | 0.7 | 3.9 |
| Visitors | 3.9 | 3.7 | 3.9 | 4.6 | 0.0 | 2.1 | 4.3 | 2.3 | 0.0 | 5.2 | 3.2 | 3.7 | 3.2 | 0.8 | 15.0 | 1.5 | 1.3 | 6.4 | 7.6 | 0.8 | 4.9 | 2.1 | 0.6 | 2.3 |
| **Location** | | | | | | | | | | | | | | | | | | | | | | | | |
| Day-room | 0.0 | 55.4 | 0.0 | 0.0 | 44.4 | 72.7 | 0.0 | 0.0 | 0.0 | 46.9 | 57.4 | 0.0 | 0.0 | 1.2 | 0.0 | 0.0 | 27.0 | 14.7 | 65.9 | 56.8 | 39.9 | 60.2 | 26.2 | 22.4 |
| Ward bay | 27.4 | 5.2 | 44.0 | 44.2 | 0.4 | 0.0 | 36.8 | 44.9 | 52.3 | 2.5 | 3.3 | 64.9 | 43.7 | 56.6 | 51.1 | 48.9 | 0.0 | 0.0 | 0.0 | 0.0 | 1.1 | 0.0 | 4.7 | 0.0 |
| In bed | 55.1 | 14.3 | 26.9 | 26.0 | 16.3 | 1.8 | 27.4 | 34.4 | 26.3 | 14.9 | 18.2 | 7.9 | 16.5 | 11.5 | 1.4 | 13.7 | 23.2 | 20.6 | 5.5 | 20.6 | 9.4 | 14.0 | 32.0 | 21.7 |

*Key:* W/C – Wholly compensatory
P/C – Partly compensatory
S/E – Supportive–educative

# Appendix IX

## LEVEL OF THERAPEUTIC CONTENT OF SELF-CARE ACTIVITIES OF PATIENTS IN THREE WARDS

| | | Brown Ward | | | White Ward | | | Red Ward | | |
|---|---|---|---|---|---|---|---|---|---|---|
| | | W/C | P/C | S/E | W/C | P/C | S/E | W/C | P/C | S/E |
| Elimination | 4 | 0.0 | 16.8 | 28.6 | 0.0 | 0.0 | 100.0 | 0.0 | 8.1 | 44.8 |
| | 3 | 1.4 | 28.4 | 5.4 | 55.5 | 62.7 | 0.0 | 15.2 | 36.4 | 29.7 |
| | 2 | 62.5 | 18.9 | 12.5 | 37.3 | 35.6 | 0.0 | 22.7 | 30.3 | 12.0 |
| | 1 | 36.1 | 35.8 | 53.6 | 7.2 | 1.7 | 0.0 | 62.1 | 25.3 | 13.5 |
| Feeding | 4 | 0.0 | 41.8 | 22.1 | 1.8 | 73.7 | 94.0 | 22.6 | 15.5 | 74.2 |
| | 3 | 27.6 | 13.9 | 20.7 | 80.7 | 9.5 | 6.0 | 0.6 | 37.6 | 0.0 |
| | 2 | 27.6 | 27.0 | 23.0 | 13.5 | 10.7 | 0.0 | 30.5 | 43.2 | 21.0 |
| | 1 | 44.7 | 17.2 | 34.3 | 4.0 | 6.2 | 0.0 | 46.3 | 3.7 | 4.8 |
| Washing | 4 | 0.0 | 12.0 | 0.0 | 1.8 | 41.2 | 76.2 | 0.0 | 0.0 | 28.0 |
| | 3 | 1.9 | 16.0 | 7.4 | 21.8 | 33.3 | 0.0 | 3.5 | 6.4 | 44.0 |
| | 2 | 25.0 | 60.0 | 29.6 | 23.6 | 13.7 | 23.8 | 16.1 | 57.4 | 20.0 |
| | 1 | 73.1 | 12.0 | 63.0 | 52.7 | 11.8 | 0.0 | 80.4 | 36.2 | 8.0 |
| Dressing | 4 | 0.0 | 0.0 | 12.8 | 0.0 | 12.8 | 100.0 | 0.0 | 0.0 | 16.1 |
| | 3 | 0.0 | 25.9 | 38.3 | 4.5 | 33.3 | 0.0 | 0.0 | 17.0 | 58.1 |
| | 2 | 41.4 | 44.4 | 2.1 | 77.3 | 53.8 | 0.0 | 46.2 | 68.1 | 25.8 |
| | 1 | 58.6 | 29.6 | 46.8 | 18.2 | 0.0 | 0.0 | 53.8 | 14.9 | 0.0 |
| Undressing | 4 | 0.0 | 0.0 | 7.1 | 0.0 | 12.5 | 100.0 | 0.0 | 28.9 | 41.2 |
| | 3 | 39.3 | 10.5 | 53.6 | 9.1 | 57.5 | 0.0 | 0.0 | 0.0 | 58.8 |
| | 2 | 14.3 | 68.4 | 21.4 | 54.6 | 30.0 | 0.0 | 0.0 | 71.1 | 0.0 |
| | 1 | 46.4 | 21.2 | 17.9 | 33.3 | 0.0 | 0.0 | 100.0 | 0.0 | 0.0 |
| Exercising | 4 | 0.0 | 0.0 | 16.9 | 0.0 | 29.6 | 0.0 | 0.0 | 24.4 | 28.4 |
| | 3 | 0.0 | 86.5 | 80.5 | 9.1 | 62.0 | 100.0 | 0.0 | 45.8 | 64.2 |
| | 2 | 0.0 | 5.4 | 1.3 | 90.9 | 7.0 | 0.0 | 0.0 | 12.9 | 3.0 |
| | 1 | 0.0 | 8.1 | 1.3 | 0.0 | 1.4 | 0.0 | 0.0 | 16.9 | 4.5 |
| Communication: | | | | | | | | | | |
| Patient-initiated | 2 | 23.5 | 79.2 | 60.0 | 0.0 | 13.3 | 40.0 | 28.3 | 4.5 | 73.3 |
| | 1 | 23.5 | 4.2 | 17.1 | 14.0 | 15.8 | 10.0 | 24.5 | 28.1 | 6.7 |
| Nurse-initiated | 2 | 32.4 | 16.7 | 20.0 | 51.8 | 46.7 | 40.0 | 32.1 | 52.8 | 20.0 |
| | 1 | 20.6 | 0.0 | 2.9 | 33.9 | 24.2 | 10.0 | 15.1 | 14.6 | 0.0 |

Note: Bathing activities were excluded because of insufficient number of observations

Key: W/C – Wholly compensatory
P/C – Partly compensatory
S/E – Supportive – educative

# References

Abdellah F G and Levine E (1979) *Better Patient Care Through Nursing Research*. New York: Macmillan.

Abdellah F G, Beland I L, Martin A and Matheney R V (1960) *Patient Centred Approaches to Nursing*. New York: Macmillan.

Abel-Smith B (1960) *A History of the Nursing Profession*. London: Heinemann.

Adams G F (1960) The third phase in geriatric medicine; design and purpose of a hosptial geriatric department. *Lancet*, 815–817.

Adams G F (1964) Clinical undertaking? *Lancet*, 1055–1058.

Adams G F (1969) *A Review of Geriatric Services in Northern Ireland Hospitals*. Belfast: Northern Ireland Hospitals Authority.

Adams G F and Cheeseman E A (1951) *Old People in Northern Ireland*. Belfast: Northern Ireland Hosptials Authority.

Adams G F and McIlwraith P L (1963) *Geriatric Nursing: A Study of the Work of Geriatric Ward Staff*. London: Oxford University Press.

Agate J (1979) *Geriatrics for Nurses and Social Workers*, 2nd edn. London: Heinemann.

Altschul A T (1972) *Patient–Nurse Interaction: A Study of Interaction Patterns in Acute Psychiatric Wards*. Edinburgh: Churchill Livingstone.

Anderson W F, Caird F I, Kennedy R D and Schwartz D (1982) *Gerontology and Geriatric Nursing*. London: Hodder and Stoughton.

Andrews J and Atkinson L (1978) Selecting equipment for elderly patients in hospital. *British Medical Journal*, 2:484.

Backscheider J E (1974) Self-care requirements, self-care capabilities and nursing systems in the diabetic nurse management clinic. *American Journal of Public Health*, **64**: 1138–1146.

Baker D E (1978) *Attitudes of Nurses to the Care of the Elderly*. Unpublished PhD thesis, University of Manchester.

Baly M E (1980) *Nursing and Social Change*, 2nd edn. London: Heinemann.

Barrowclough F and Pinel C (1979) *Geriatric Care for Nurses*. London: Heinemann.

de Beauvoir (1973) *Old Age*. London: Andrew Deutsch.

Becker H S, Greer B, Hughes E C and Strauss A C (1961) *Boys in White*. Chicago: University of Chicago Press.

Bergman R (1983) Understanding the patient in all his human needs. *Journal of Advanced Nursing*, **8**: 185–190.

Bloch D (1975) Evaluation of nursing care in terms of process and outcome: issues in research and quality assurance. *Nursing Research*, **24**(4): 256–263.

Boore J R P (1978) *Prescription for Recovery: The Effect of Pre-operative Preparation of Surgical Patients on Post-operative Stress, Recovery and Infection*. London: Royal College of Nursing.

Brand J (1975) The politics of social indicators. *British Journal of Sociology*, **XXVI**: 78–90.

Brayfield A H and Rothe H F (1951) An index of job satisfaction. *Journal of Applied Psychology*, **35**: 307–311.

British Geriatric Society (1976) Memorandum. British Geriatric Society, Burnley Sunley House, 60 Pitcairn Road, Mitcham.

British Geriatric Society and Royal College of Nursing (1975) *Improving Geriatric Care in Hospital*. London: Royal College of Nursing.

British Medical Association (1976) *Care of the Elderly. Report of the Working Party on Services for the Elderly*. London: British Medical Association.

Brocklehurst J C (1973) Incontinence in the elderly. *Nursing Mirror*, **136**: 30–32.

Brocklehurst J C (ed.) (1975) *Geriatric Care in Advanced Societies*. London: MTP.

Brocklehurst J C (ed.) (1978) *Textbook of Geriatric Medicine and Gerontology*. Edinburgh: Churchill Livingstone.

Bunge M (1975) What is a quality of life indicator? *Social Indicator Research*, **2**: 65–69.

Burnside I M (1976) *Nursing and the Aged*. New York: McGraw-Hill.

Callaghan A (1968) *Nursing Duties in Geriatric Wards G1, G2 and G3 at Warrington General Hospital*. Liverpool: Liverpool Regional Hospital Board.

Carley M (1981) *Social Measurement and Social Indicators. Issues of Policy and Theory*. London: George Allen and Unwin.

Carlisle E (1972) The conceptual structure of social indicators. In: *Social Indicators and Social Policy*, Shonfield A and Shaw S (eds.). London: Heinemann Educational Books.

Carnevali D L and Patrick M (1979) *Nursing Management for the Elderly*. New York: J B Lippincott.

Chalmers G L (1980) *Caring for the Elderly Sick*. Tunbridge Wells: Pitman Medical.

Chisholm M K (1977) The nurse's responsibility when caring for the elderly. *Nursing Times*, **73**: 1509–1510.

Clark J (1982) Development of models and theories on the concept of nursing. *Journal of Advanced Nursing*, **7**: 129–134.

Clark M (1973) Advance the advanced: the role and work of nurses in a multidisciplinary geriatric team. *Nursing Times*, **69**: 1452–1453.

Coakley D (ed.) (1982) *Establishing a Geriatric Service*. London: Croom Helm.

Cruise V J (1978) Better geriatric care – making it happen. *Nursing Times,* **74**: 1503–1564.

Dartington T, Jones P and Miller E (1974) *Geriatric Hospital Care.* London: Tavistock Institute of Human Relations.

Dent R V (1977) Geriatric care in hospital. *Nursing Times,* **73**: 1507–1509.

Department of Health and Social Security (1969) *Report of the Committee of Enquiry into Allegations of Ill Treatment of Patients and Other Irregularities at Ely Hospital, Cardiff.* Cmnd 3975. London: HMSO.

Department of Health and Social Security (1971) *Report of the Farleigh Hospital Committee of Enquiry.* Cmnd 4557. London: HMSO.

Department of Health and Social Security (1972a) *Report of the Committee of Enquiry into Whittingham Hospital.* Cmnd 4861. London: HMSO.

Department of Health and Social Security (1972b) *Report the of Committee on Nursing* (Chairman: A. Briggs). London: HMSO

Department of Health and Social Security (1977) *Priorities in the Health and Social Services – The Way Forward.* London: HMSO.

Department of Health and Social Security (1978) *A Happier Old Age: A Discussion Document on Elderly People in our Society.* London: HMSO.

Dickoff J and James P (1968) A theory of theories: a position paper. *Nursing Research,* **17**: 197–203.

Dickoff J, James P and Wiedenbach E (1968) Theory in a practice discipline – Part 1. Practice oriented theory. *Nursing Research,* **17**: 415–435.

Dolan J, Shanahan D and Whitehead A (1972) Growth of a day hospital. *Nursing Mirror,* **135**: 22–24.

Eldridge J (ed.) (1971) *Max Weber: The Interpretation of Social Reality.* London: Michael Joseph.

Evans G, Hodkinson H M and Mezey A G (1971) The elderly sick: who looks after them? *Lancet,* **2**: 539–541.

Evers H R (1981a) Tender loving care? – patients and nurses in geriatric wards. In: *Care of the Aging,* Copp L A (ed.). Edinburgh: Churchill Livingstone.

Evers H R (1981b) Multidisciplinary teams in geriatric wards: myth or reality. *Journal of Advanced Nursing,* **6**: 205–214.

Evers H R (1982a) Key issues in nursing practice: ward management – I. *Nursing Times* Occasional Paper, **78**: 25–26.

Evers H R (1982b) Key issues in nursing practice: ward management – II *Nursing Times* Occasional Paper,**78**: 25–26.

Exton-Smith A N (1962) Progressive patient care in geriatrics. *Lancet,* **1**: 260–262.

Finlay O E (1982) Designing a chair to suit the needs of the elderly. *Therapy,* June 1982.

Fleming I, Barrowclough C and Whitmore B (1983) The constructional approach. *Nursing Mirror,* **156**: 21–23.

Fox D (1982) *Fundamentals of Research in Nursing,* 4th edn. Norwalk: Appleton-Century-Crofts.

Fretwell J E (1978) *Socialisation of Nurses: Teaching and Learning in Hospital Wards.* Unpublished PhD thesis, University of Warwick.

Goddard H (1953) *The Work of Nurses in Hospital Wards, Report of a Job Analysis.* Oxford: The Nuffield Provincial Hospital Trust.

Goddard H (1963) *Work Measurement as a Basis for Calculating Nursing Establishments, An Analytical Study.* Leeds: Leeds Regional Hospital Board.

Grant N (1979) *Time to Care. A Method of Calculating Nursing Workload Based on Individualised Patient Care.* London: Royal College of Nursing.

Griffin A P (1980) Philosophy and nursing. *Journal of Advanced Nursing.* 5: 261–272.

Griffin A P (1983) A philosophical analysis of caring in nursing. *Journal of Advanced Nursing,* 8: 289–295.

Halliburton P M and Wright W B (1974) Towards better geriatric care. *Social Work Today,* 5: 107–108.

Hardy L K (1982) Nursing models and research – a restricting view? *Journal of Advanced Nursing,* 7: 447–457.

Hardy M E (1974) Theories: components, development, evaluation. *Nursing Research,* 23: 100–107.

Hayward J (1975) *Information – A Prescription against Pain.* London: Royal College of Nursing.

Henderson V (1966) *Basic Principles of Nursing.* London: ICN.

Henderson V (1980) Preserving the essence of nursing in a technological age. *Journal of Advanced Nursing,* 5: 240–260.

Hirschfeld M (1979) Research in nursing gerontology. *Journal of Advanced Nursing,* 4: 621–626.

Hirschfeld M (1983) Home care versus institutionalisation: family caregiving and senile brain disease. *International Journal of Nursing Studies,* 20: 23–32.

Hobman D (1982) Grey areas. *Times Health Supplement,* 23: 17.

Hockey L (1976) *Women in Nursing: A Descriptive Study.* London: Hodder and Stoughton.

Hockey L (1977) Indicators in nursing research with emphasis on social indicators. *Journal of Advanced Nursing,* 2: 239–250.

Hodkinson H M (1975) *An Outline of Geriatrics,* 1st edn. London: Academic Press.

Hodkinson H M (1981) *An Outline of Geriatrics.* London: Academic Press.

Hodkinson H M and Jeffreys P M (1972) Making hospital geriatrics work. *British Medical Journal,* 4: 536–539.

Hodkinson I and Hodkinson H M (1981) The long-term stay patient. *Gerontology,* 27: 167–172.

Hogstel M O (1981) *Nursing Care of the Older Adult.* New York: John Wiley and Sons.

Hooper J (1981a) Geriatric patients and nurse learners' attitudes. *Nursing Times (Occasional Paper),* 77: 34–40.

Hooper J (1981b) Geriatric patients and nurse learners' attitudes. *Nursing Times (Occasional Paper),* 77: 41–43.

Horrocks P (1979) The case for geriatric medicine as an age-related specialty. In: *Recent Advances in Geriatric Medicine,* Isaacs B (ed.). Edinburgh: Churchill Livingstone.

Horrocks P (1983) Hospital treatment of the elderly – new directions. *British Journal of Geriatric Nursing*, **3**: 3–5.

Howell T H (1972) Staffing questions in a new geriatric unit. *Hospital and Health Services Review*, **68**: 17–19.

Hunt J M and Marks-Maran D J (1980) *Nursing Care Plans. The Nursing Process at Work*. Aylesbury: HM + M.

Inman U (1975) *Towards a Theory of Nursing Care*. London: Royal College of Nursing.

Irvine R E, Bagnall M K and Smith B J (1978) *The Older Patient: A textbook of Geriatrics*, 3rd edn. London: Hodder and Stoughton.

Isaacs B (1973) Treatment of 'irremediable' elderly patients. *British Medical Journal*, **3**: 526–528.

Jeffreys M (1978) The elderly in society. In: *Textbook of Geriatric Medicine and Gerontology*, Brocklehurst J (ed.). Edinburgh: Churchill Livingstone.

Johnson M (1983) Some aspects of the relation between theory and research in nursing. *Journal of Advanced Nursing*, **8**: 21–28.

Johnson M L (1978) Nursing auxiliaries and nurse professionalization. *Nursing Times*, **74**: 313–317.

Joseph L S (1980) Self-care and the nursing process. *Nursing Clinics of North America*, **15**: 131–143.

Kemp J (1978) The elderly: a challenge to nursing. *Nursing Times*, **74**: 198–199.

Kerlinger F N (1973) *Foundations in Behavioural Research*, 2nd edn. New York: Holt, Rinehart and Winston.

King I M (1981) *A Theory of Nursing: Systems, Concepts, Process*. New York: John Wiley and Sons.

Kitson A L (1983) *A Study of Geriatric Wards, Their Patients and Nursing Staff in Northern Ireland*. Coleraine: New University of Ulster.

Kitson A L (1984) *Steps Toward the Indentification and Development of Nursing's Therapeutic Function in the Care of the Hospitalized Elderly*. DPhil thesis, School of Social Science, New University of Ulster.

Land K C (1971) On the definition of social indicators. *The American Sociologist*, **6**: 322–325.

Levin L, Katz A and Holst E (1979) *Self Care: Lay Initiatives in Health*, 2nd edn. New York: Prodist.

Lewis J A (1966) Reflections on self. In: *Psychiatric Nursing, Vol. 1, Developing Psychiatric Nursing Skills*, Mereness D (ed.), New York: NMC Brown.

Little D E and Carnevali D L (1969) *Nursing Care Planning*. Philadelphia: J B Lippincott.

Luker K A (1981) An overview of evaluation research in nursing. *Journal of Advanced Nursing*, **6**: 87–94.

McFarlane E A (1980) Nursing theory: the comparison of four theoretical proposals. *Journal of Advanced Nursing*, **5**: 3–19.

McFarlane J (1970) *The Proper Study of the Nurse*. London: Royal College of Nursing.

McFarlane J (1976) A charter for caring. *Journal of Advanced Nursing*, **1**: 187–196.

McHugh J C and Chughtai M A (1975) The importance of teamwork in geriatric care. *Nursing Times,* **71**: 140–142.

MacIntyre S (1977) Old age as a social problem. In: *Health Care and Health Knowledge,* Dingwall R, Heath C, Reid M and Stacey M (eds.). London: Croom Helm.

McLeod F R (1976) *Geriatric Care.* Aylesbury: HM + M.

Magid S and Rhys Hearn C (1980) Some characteristics of geriatric patients in hospital wards. *International Journal of Nursing Studies,* **17**(2): 97–106.

Mangan P (1982) The right of choice. *British Journal of Geriatric Nursing,* **2**: 8–9.

Mayers M (1978) *A Systematic Approach to Nursing Care Plans.* New York: Appleton-Century Crofts.

Miller A E (1978) *Evaluation of the Care Provided for Patients with Dementia in Six Hospital Wards.* Unpublished MSc thesis, University of Manchester.

Miller E J and Gwynne G V (1972) *A Life Apart: A Pilot Study of Residential Institutions for the Physically Handicapped and the Young Chronic Sick.* London: Tavistock.

Milligan P K (1973) Progressive patient care. *Nursing Mirror,* **137**: 34–38.

Murray R B, Huelskoetter M and O'Driscoll D (1980) *The Nursing Process in Later Maturity.* New York: Prentice Hall.

Norman A J (1980) *Rights and Risk.* London: The National Corporation for the Care of Old People.

Norton D (1954) A challenge to nursing. *Nursing Times,* **50**: 1253–1258.

Norton D (1965) Nursing in geriatrics. *Gerontologia Clinica,* **7**: 57–60.

Norton D (1967) *Hospitals of the Long Stay Patients.* Oxford: Pergamon Press.

Norton D (1970) *By Accident or Design?* Edinburgh: Churchill Livingstone.

Norton D (1977) Geriatric nursing – what it is and what it is not. *Nursing Times,* **73**: 1622–1623.

Norton D (1981) Let there be no misunderstanding. *British Journal of Geriatrics,* **1**, editorial.

Norton D, McLaren R and Exton-Smith A N (1962) *An Investigation of Geriatric Nursing Problems in Hospital.* London: National Corporation for the Care of Old People, reprinted in 1976 by Churchill Livingstone.

Norwich H S (1980) A study of nursing care in geriatric hospitals. *Nursing Times,* **76**: 292–295.

Nursing Development Conference Group (1973) *Concept Formalization in Nursing.* Boston: Little, Brown and Co.

O'Rawe A M (1982) Self-neglect – a challenge for nursing. *Nursing Times,* **78**: 1932–1936.

Orem D (1971) *Nursing: Concepts of Practice.* New York: McGraw Hill.

Orem D (1980) *Nursing: Concepts of Practice,* 2nd edn. New York: McGraw Hill.

Orton H D (1979) *Ward Learning Climate and Student Nurse Response.* Unpublished MPhil thesis, Sheffied City Polytechnic.

Parnell J N and Naylor R (1973) *Home for the Weekend − Back on Monday.*
London: Queen's Institute for District Nursing.

Pathy S (1982) Operational Policies. In: *Establishing a Geriatric Service,*
Coakley D (ed.). London: Croom Helm.

Pembrey S (1980) *The Ward Sister − Key to Nursing: A Study of the
Organization of Individualized Nursing.* London: Royal College of
Nursing.

Peplau H E (1952) *Interpersonal Relations in Nursing.* New York: Putnam.

Pinel C (1976) Geriatrics as a specialty. *Nursing Times,* **72**: 1601−1603.

Rands V (1972) Geriatric nursing services. *Nursing Times,* **68**: 1054−1057.

Redfern S (1979) *The Charge Nurse: Job Attitudes and Occupation Stability.*
Unpublished PhD thesis, University of Aston, Birmingham.

Redfern S (1981) Evaluating care of the elderly: a British perspective.
In: Care of the Aging, Copp L A (ed.). Edinburgh: Churchill Livingstone.

Reid E (1981) Nursing care of the aged: an overview of education,
research and practice in England and Wales. *Journal of Gerontological
Nursing,* **7**: 733−738.

Rhys Hearn C (1979a) Staffing geriatric wards: trials of a 'package' − 1.
*Nursing Times* Occasional Paper, **75**: 45−48.

Rhys Hearn C (1979b) Staffing geriatric wards: trials of a 'package' − 2.
*Nursing Times* Occasional Paper, **75**: 52.

Rhys Hearn C and Howard J (1980) The relationship of nursing needs,
resources and standards in geriatric wards. In: *Management Services and
the Nurse,* Department of Health and Social Security unpublished
report. London: DHSS.

Rhys Hearn C and Potts D (1978) The effect of patients' individual
characteristics upon activity times for items of nursing care.
*International Journal of Nursing,* **15**: 23−30.

Riehl J P and Roy C (1980) *Conceptual Models for Nursing Practice,* 2nd edn.
New York: Appleton-Century-Crofts.

Robb B (1967) *Sans Everything.* London: Nelson.

Roy C (1980) The Roy Adaptation Model. In: *Conceptual Models for Nursing
Practice,* 2nd edn. Riehl J P and Roy C eds. New York:
Appleton-Century-Crofts.

Royal College of Physicians of London (1977) *Report of the Working Party
on the Medical Care of the Elderly.* London: Royal College of Physicians.

Rudd T N (1954) *The Nursing of the Elderly Sick. A Practical Handbook for
Geriatric Nursing.* London: Faber.

Savage B, Widdowson T and Wright T (1979) Improving the care of the
elderly. In: *Innovation in Patient Care: An Action Research Study of Change
in a Psychiatric Hospital,* Towell D and Harries C (eds.). London: Croom
Helm.

Scottish Home and Health Department (1967) *Nurses' Work in Hospitals in
the North-Eastern Region,* Scottish Health Service Studies no. 3.
Edinburgh: SHHD.

Sharmann I M (1972) Nutrition for the elderly. *Nursing Mirror,* **134**:
43−45.

Sheldon J H (1948) *The Social Medicine of Old Age.* London: Oxford University Press.

Silverman D (1970) *The Theory of Organizations.* London: Heinemann.

Skeet M H (1970) *Home from Hospital.* London: The Dan Mason Nursing Research Committee.

Skeet M H (1982) A nurse for all settings. *British Journal of Geriatric Nursing,* **1**: 15–19.

Smith L (1982) Models of nursing as the basis for curriculum development: some rationales and implications. *Journal of Advanced Nurisng,* **7**: 117–127.

Stevens B J (1979) *Nursing Theory.* Boston: Little, Brown and Company.

Stockwell F (1972) *The Unpopular Patient.* London: Royal College of Nursing.

Storrs A M F (1975) *Geriatric Nursing.* London: Baillière Tindall.

Storrs A M F (1982) What is care? *British Journal of Geriatric Nursing,* **1**: 12–14.

Strauss A, Schatzman L, Erlich D, Bucher R and Sabshin M (1963) The hospital and its negotiated order. In: *The Hospital in Modern Society,* Friedson E (ed.). Glencoe: Free Press.

Tiffany R (1979) Mobilizing skills. *Journal of Advanced Nursing,* **4**: 3–8.

Tinker A (1981) *The Elderly in Modern Society.* London: Longman.

Topliss E P (1973) Staffing in a geriatric hospital. *Health and Social Services Journal,* **83**: 202–204.

Towell D (1975) *Understanding Psychiatric Nursing.* London: Royal College of Nursing.

Towell D (1979) A 'social systems' approach to research and change in nursing care. *International Journal of Nursing Studies,* **16**: 111–121.

Travelbee J (1977) *Interpersonal Aspects of Nursing,* 2nd edn. Philadelphia: F A David

Trott C (1970) Personal clothing for patients. *The Hospital,* **68**: 111–113.

Uys L R (1980) Towards the development of an operational definition of the concept 'therapeutic use of self'. *International Journal of Nursing Studies,* **17**: 175–180.

Wade B and Snaith P (1981) The assessment of patients' need for nursing care on geriatric wards. *International Journal of Nursing Studies,* **18**: 261–271.

Watson F (1982) Quality of life in old age. *Nursing Times,* Community Outlook, **78**: 309–310, 314, 317–318.

Wells T (1980) *Problems in Geriatric Nursing Care. A Study of Nurses' Problems in Care of Old People in Hospitals.* Edinburgh: Churchill Livingstone.

West J (1976) Modern Geriatric Unit – Tolworth Hospital. *Nursing Mirror,* **142**: 67–69.

White R (1978) *Social Change and the Development of the Nursing Profession. A Study of the Poor Law Nursing Service, 1848–1948.* London: Kingston.

Whitmore D (1970) *Work Study and Related Management Services,* 2nd edn. London: Heinemann.

Williamson J D and Danaher K (1978) *Self-care in Health.* London: Croom Helm.

Yura H and Walsh M (1973) *The Nursing Process.* New York: Appleton-Century-Crofts.

Yurick A G, Robb S S, Spier B E and Ebert N J (1980) *The Aged Person and the Nursing Process.* New York: Appleton-Century-Crofts.

# Further reading

Adams G F (1952), Long-stay accommodation for the elderly irremediable patient. *Ulster Medical Journal,* **XXI,** 177–184.

Davies A and Snaith P A (1980) The social behaviour of geriatric patients at mealtimes. *Age and Ageing,* **9:** 93–99.

Department of Health and Social Security (1972c) *Minimum Standards in Geriatric Hospitals and Departments.* Cmnd D.S.95/72. London: HMSO.

Department of Health and Social Security (1981a) *Health Building Note 37, Hospital Accommodation for Elderly People.* London: HMSO.

Department of Health and Social Security (1981b) *Report of a Study on the Respctive Roles of the General Acute and Geriatric Sectors of the Care of the Elderly Hospital Patient.* London: HMSO.

Department of Health and Social Services (NI), Research and Intelligence Unit. (1972) *Health and Personal Social Services Statistics for Northern Ireland.* Belfast: HMSO.

Department of Health and Social Services (NI) (1975a) *Report on the Development of Hospital Services in the Area of the Northern Health and Social Services Board,* vol. 2. Belfast: HMSO.

Department of Health and Social Services (NI) Works Unit. (1975b) *A Report in Collaboration with the National Building Agency.* Belfast: HMSO.

Department of Health and Social Services (NI) (1981) *Post Sixty-Five, Who Cares? A Report on Health and Personal Social Services for Elderly People in Northern Ireland.* Belfast: HMSO.

Ebersole P and Hess P (1982) *Towards Healthy Ageing. Human Needs and Nursing Response.* St. Louis: C V Mosby.

Goffman E (1968) *Asylums.* Harmondsworth: Penguin.

Goffman E (1968) *Stigma.* Harmondsworth: Penguin.

Norton D (1975) The ergonomically organized environment. *Hospital Equipment and Supplies,* **21**: 40–42.

Norton D (1978) Equipment Fit for Purpose. *Nursing Times,* Occasional Paper, **74**: 73–76.

Riehl J P and Roy C (1974) *Conceptual Models for Nursing Practice.* New York: Appleton-Century-Crofts.

Scottish Home and Health Department (1970) *Geriatric Accommodation Report.* Edinburgh: SHHD.

Scottish Hospital Centre (1974) *Ward Conversion for Geriatric Patients.* Edinburgh: SHC.

Siegel S (1956) *Nonparametric Statistics for the Behavioural Sciences.* International Student Edition. New York: McGraw Hill.

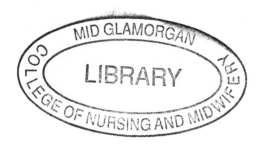